Wellness and Harmony

A THIRTY-DAY JOURNEY
FOR HOSPICE CAREGIVERS

John A. Love

WESTBOW
PRESS®
A DIVISION OF THOMAS NELSON
& ZONDERVAN

WestBow Press books may be ordered through booksellers or by contacting:

WestBow Press
A Division of Thomas Nelson & Zondervan
1663 Liberty Drive
Bloomington, IN 47403
www.westbowpress.com
1 (866) 928-1240

Front Cover: Red Wing Pond, Brown County, Indiana
Photograph by Lynn Love

ISBN: 978-1-9736-6736-0 (sc)
ISBN: 978-1-9736-6735-3 (e)

Library of Congress Control Number: 2019908584

Print information available on the last page.

WestBow Press rev. date: 05/6/2020

Through those who serve the dying – through their tireless work, selfless devotion, and endless gifts of kindness – we see the hands and heart of God.

CONTENTS

PRELUDE

Humanity is the collective result of individual connections and interactions. Life typically begins with a natural mother and child bond. Very quickly, other family members are added to the mix. These foundational relationships prepare us for what lies ahead. While growing up, we develop friendships. Some are close and lasting, while others are shallow and fleeting. Some are loving, others are not. Either way, we learn from them. Adult connections are often forged among like-minded people who share things in common: living on the same street, visiting the same park, enjoying the same hobby, working for the same employer, and so on. In total, these relationships not only shape our identity, they influence how we perceive the world.

By design, life is dynamic. And since we don't live in a vacuum, a host of local, national, and world events capture our attention. We are repulsed by violent crimes, even when they happen in another city. We are troubled by discrimination, regardless of where it occurs. We're disturbed by global oppression and corrupt governments. We're dismayed by enslavement and exploitation. We are appalled by war and genocide. And we are alarmed by poverty, disease, pain, and suffering – whether it's found in a faraway country, or in our own neighborhood.

If you scan the news, then you're probably reading detailed accounts of tragic accidents. You're probably listening to graphic descriptions of global catastrophes and acts of terror. Perhaps you're also keeping up with politics. And if that's the case, then you're likely to read about a hopelessly divided America. It's hard to withstand these endless waves of negativity. Eventually, you become entangled in a web of despair. You start to believe that the world is falling apart, and humanity is on the brink of extinction.

Then, you go to work – to an environment that has its own elements of pain. You build trust-based relationships with your hospice patients, knowing that these treasured connections end much too soon. You see a perpetual queue of unfamiliar faces replacing the ones you had grown to love, the ones who had smiled each time they saw you. All of this happens with so little time to grieve, so little time to heal. Is it any wonder that you frequently feel sad and heartbroken? When looking in a mirror, are you really surprised to see signs of fatigue and depletion?

Those who serve the dying confront high-acuity challenges each and every day. What's more, hospice workers face the very real risk of developing burnout – a debilitating lethargy that can prematurely end a promising career. Although newly hired caregivers are eager to start, research indicates that doubts begin to surface somewhere between six and twelve months on the job. Still, there's good news. For the same study shows that by the time hospice workers reach their two-year anniversary, outlooks are improving. Caregivers are learning how to cope and persevere. Gradually, the work becomes more and more meaningful, more and more rewarding. In due time, hospice care is seen as a viable career, and the future is bright.

Those who provide direct patient care are, of course, part of an interdisciplinary team. Therefore, when a caregiver leaves, each teammate is affected. And any loss of continuity will, on some level, impact workers and patients alike. To be honest, staff turnover not only strains hospice resources, it deflates morale as well. So if you're a newcomer, here's the key: Acquire the coping tools needed to carry you into your second year and beyond. And if you're a seasoned staff member, remain vigilant. Be committed to practicing holistic self-care right along with your coworkers who've just finished orientation.

It is hoped that *Wellness and Harmony* will inform, uplift, and inspire you – whether you're an enthusiastic beginner or a proud veteran. To that end, the material is thought provoking, yet reassuring. Much of the content is spiritual in nature, but not religious. Maybe the lessons will help you perceive the world a bit differently, and that alone can be wonderfully energizing.

With this backdrop in place, it's time to begin your thirty-day journey. Each chapter explores a new topic. You'll find helpful tips, practical interventions, and quiet reflections. Think of this endeavor as an opportunity for introspection. Therefore, allow the pathway to turn inward. By looking deeply into your heart, you'll become a more compassionate and effective caregiver, a more nurturing and attentive parent, a more loving and supportive partner, and a more fulfilled and grateful person. And yes, an introspective journey will strengthen your most important relationship: the one you have with God.

As you practice the recommended self-care tips, your calmness and confidence will grow. And as your inner strength blossoms, your faith and trust will grow as well. Though your first steps may be small and tentative, they will be empowering nonetheless. Each subsequent stride will take you closer to work-life excellence. Be assured that your pathway will ultimately lead to a healthier, happier life. Finally, bear in mind that every triumphant journey begins with a humble first step.

★★★

Nestled among the mountains of Europe, an abbey sits patiently, unaffected by changing seasons or passing time. Towering walls have thwarted all enemies, while spartan rooms have welcomed all strangers. Songbirds grace the abbey's cemetery, the peaceful resting place for generations of monks. Today, the men in this cloistered community will worship and work, study and contemplate. They will eat and sleep, pray and meditate. Most of these activities will unfold in vowed silence. Yet there's seldom a lack of communication. Seated at the dinner table, a monk – at just the right moment, and without a prompting word or gesture – will pass the salt to his neighbor.

The abbey is a sanctuary for those who choose to live there. When a monk is sad, his brothers uplift him. When a monk is sick, his brothers nurture him. And when a monk is dying, his brothers comfort him. Long ago, this same kind of love and devotion inspired the anam cara – the soul friend. These highly skilled caregivers maintained vigils for the dying. Organic poultices, herbal tonics, and natural analgesics were used to alleviate pain. The anam cara created a sacred space in which to listen and affirm. Soul friends offered gentle touch and simpatico breathing. They recited liturgies. They chanted and prayed. And unknowingly, these dedicated men and women were planting the seeds of present-day hospice care.

★★★

Spiritual teachers have observed that an unhealed healer helps no one.

★★★

DAY ONE

CREATING A COVENANT

There are two great days in life – the day we are born,
and the day we discover why. *William Barclay*

★★★

When living intentionally, you are proactive instead of reactive. It means taking charge of your life, making choices, and being accountable for the consequences of your choices. It also satisfies the human need to maintain a sense of control. What's more, intentionality is empowering because it prevents you from perceiving yourself as a victim.

In keeping with this premise, there are three reasons to write a Covenant. First, a Covenant defines your life's purpose and intentionality. This involves a contemplative process – an examination of your beliefs and intentions followed by a decision as to which ones to keep, which ones to discard, and which ones to change. Secondly, you are making your beliefs and intentions explicit by documenting them. In truth, you cannot live intentionally unless your goals and values are in writing. Finally, a Covenant is a contract between yourself and God, an agreement that demonstrates your desire to live a meaningful life.

By design, a Covenant provides you with direction and motivation in achieving your full potential, both personal and professional. It should be written in an active and purposeful voice, and it should offer vision and clarity. A Covenant must describe your best-self, the person you hope to become; and it must identify the pathway needed to attain this goal. A Covenant acknowledges that you are an essential part of something much larger and grander. Lastly, a Covenant directs you to seek self-approval, rather than approval from others.

An empowering Covenant ...

Represents the deepest and best within you. It comes from a connection with your inner-self.

Declares your one-of-a-kind talents and expresses your unique ability to serve others.

Is transcendent. It is based on a foundation of service, and for a purpose higher than self.

Includes fulfillment in physical, social, mental, and spiritual dimensions.

Is based on principles that produce quality of life results.

Includes morals, ethics, values, and vision.

Embraces character and competence, who you want to be and what you want to do.

Includes all of the important roles in your life.

Represents a balance of personal, professional, and spiritual growth.

Embraces family and community responsibilities.

Is written to inspire you, not to impress someone else.

Speaks to you in a way that touches your heart.

Start with a period of reflection.

Answer the following five questions:

What is your purpose for being alive?

What do you want to improve?

What are your unfulfilled dreams?

What is truly important to you?

What are your greatest strengths?

What is your mission?

Now, review your answers.

What do they tell you about yourself?

Where are you aligned with your values and principles?

Where are you out of alignment?

What adjustments can you make?

Next, create your vision for the future by finishing the following sentences.

It is my goal to live ...

It is my goal to work ...

It is my goal to continue ...

It is my goal to love ...

It is my goal to be ...

It is my goal to believe ...

It is my goal to promote ...

It is my goal to strive ...

It is my goal to seek ...

Now, write your Covenant and hold nothing back!

★★★

Keep your Covenant in a safe, but accessible place. Refer to it whenever you lose sight of your goals or become frustrated with your personal or professional pathway. Read your Covenant from top to bottom at least three times a year in order to evaluate your progress. During these reviews, don't be too hard on yourself. Be sure to identify and celebrate the areas where you're making progress. And because it's a living document, you can revise your goals from time to time. A Covenant is, ultimately, a promise founded on love. So as you strive to meet the high standards of your Covenant, you are being true to yourself, and you are honoring God as well. Remain committed to your mission. Expect nothing more, but accept nothing less.

★★★

DAY TWO

MINDFULNESS

> When you settle into the present moment, beauty and
> wonder appear right before your eyes. *Thich Nhat Hanh*

★★★

Currently heralded by wellness experts, life coaches, and counselors, mindfulness principles and methods were first taught in India as early as 500 BC. Old World mystics fully understood the benefits of mindfulness and, interestingly, its modern-day foundation remains largely unchanged. Mindfulness concepts are easy to grasp, but difficult to master. Still, even a rudimentary understanding and application will yield desirable outcomes. Mindfulness skills promote greater awareness and focus both at work and at home. And yes, mindfulness techniques enhance overall health and well-being. In truth, mindfulness and wellness are partners – connected, yet distinctly individual. Mindfulness is the pathway; wellness is the destination.

Secular therapists embrace mindfulness because it helps people let go of negativity. Moreover, it demands that they stop making judgments. That said, mindfulness wields its greatest power within a spiritual context. Wise teachers have pointed out that we are spiritual beings on a human journey. And mindfulness, at its core, is spiritual work. It nourishes the soul.

It's helpful to have a working definition of mindfulness, a foundation to build on. But the definition must be reasonably simple to understand, integrate, and apply. To that end: *Mindfulness is a purposeful and nonjudgmental awareness of the ever-unfolding present moment.* Consider reading this definition again. Reflect on the words, and perhaps memorize them – for they are the beginning of a new chapter in your life.

The purposeful aspect of mindfulness is making an intentional choice to focus on the here and now, to fully experience what is happening *this moment*. It requires mental discipline and resolve. And like most things, the only way to sharpen your mindfulness skills is to practice them. Incidentally, the favorite excuse for *not* practicing mindfulness is: I'm too busy. But is that actually true? Are you too busy to take a shower in the morning? Are you too busy to eat a granola bar at some point in your day? Of course you have time – or can make time – for these things. But when you *are* showering, what are your thoughts? Are you worried that rush hour traffic will make you late for the team meeting? And when you *are* eating a snack, what's going through your head? Are you wondering if your patient, Mr. Jones will be as combative as the last time you saw him?

Here's what you should remember. Mindfulness is focusing entirely on the task that's unfolding. Too often, we're on autopilot. We sleepwalk through life. We can't remember if we brushed our teeth or swallowed our vitamins. On the expressway, we might drive right past the exit we want to take. As John Lennon mused, life is what happens while we're busy making other plans.

The nonjudgmental aspect of mindfulness is maintaining an awareness of your thoughts. And going a step further, try to avoid forming opinions on what is happening. Try to avoid labeling things good or bad, desirable or undesirable. Simply accept what *is*. After all, since you can't change what *is*, there's nothing gained by resisting it. As you face what *is*, simply bless it and let it go. The objective, then, is to monitor your thoughts with the purpose of dismissing negative opinions and judgments as they arise. And as you learn to let go of negativity, your inner peace will grow exponentially.

★★★

Mindfulness includes intentionality; it includes monitoring your thoughts and feelings.

★★★

Naturally, some experiences are more pleasant than others. But ultimately, you must take ownership of your thoughts.

★★★

Research has shown that it's actually impossible for the human brain to multitask. In other words, multitasking is doing several things poorly at the same time.

★★★

This one moment, **now**, is forever constant. Regardless of what happens, it happens **now**. No matter when you look at a clock, it is always **now**. Resistance is futile; and since there's no escape, why not make **now** your friend? By doing so, you will feel more at home, more at ease. Embracing **now** is an empowering choice. Then, rather than trying to manipulate life, perhaps you will allow events to unfold at their own pace. And rather than judging life, perhaps you will accept that what *is* happening is exactly what should be happening **now**. When you're engaged in a routine task, like washing dishes, what's more important: the *doing*, or the finishing? What do you value more: *this* moment, or a future moment? Is **now** just a nuisance to endure, just a barrier to overcome?

The past can only be remembered **now**. The future can only be anticipated **now**. Or think of it this way. The past unfolded in the **now** that was then, and the future will unfold in the **now** that's to come. Are you missing a sense of satisfaction and achievement **now**, while hoping for a better feeling later? Have you forgotten that the future never arrives, except as the present moment? **Now** is the only time you can live, the only time you can make the world a better place. When living in the **now**, there's no room for creating imaginary problems. Life is simpler, and it's perceived with greater clarity.

★★★

Your ego wants you to miss today's joy while waiting for tomorrow's happiness.

★★★

The past is not here now, so it can no longer harm you. The future is not yet here, so it cannot harm you now. You are safe in this present moment.

★★★

Make up your mind to drink fully from the cup of life. Then, don't settle for anything less!

★★★

Your mindfulness creates a sacred space at the patient's bedside. And within that sacred space, you build a holy relationship — a selfless connection founded on trust, and free of hidden agendas. In that mindful presence, your care giving is a spiritual endeavor.

★★★

When you are truly present for your patients, you are offering the respect they deserve. And when you are fully focused on their care, patients notice your heartfelt commitment, and they appreciate it.

★★★

During your bedside care, let go of negative thoughts and judgments. Be wholly immersed in the tasks at hand. Be kind, attentive, and compassionate in all that you think, say, and do.

★★★

If you wish, you can reach out to God for guidance at the beginning of every workday. You can ask to arrive at just the right place, at just the right moment. And you can ask God for inspiration — for the insight to say and do whatever is most helpful for each patient you visit.

★★★

In your personal life, mindfulness strengthens relationships with friends and family members, and it promotes much needed rest and renewal. Therefore, practicing mindfulness at home reduces the risk of burnout at work; and by practicing mindfulness at work, you develop the skills needed to enjoy quality time with loved ones at home.

★★★

Purposeful attention, awareness, and appreciation are vital elements of mindfulness. Mindfulness is an experience that joins thoughts, actions, sensations, and emotions. Take a look at two examples.

Eating an Orange ...

Examine it visually, notice it's shape, it's color, and it's dimpled skin.

Hold it, touch it, and feel it's texture.

Smell it as you peel the skin.

Separate the orange into two halves and listen closely for the sound of breaking fibers.

Break open a single slice of the orange.

Press it to your lips and feel its moisture.

Place it on your tongue.

Taste it and savor its flavor.

Feel what it's like to chew the orange.

Notice how the juice squirts inside your mouth.

Swallow a bite and follow the sensation of the orange as it passes your throat and gradually descends all the way down to your stomach. Eating is a delightful experience if you choose to make it so.

Taking a Shower ...

Turn on the water and listen to the sound it makes.

Place your hand in the water and feel the stinging droplets.

Keeping your hand in the water, adjust the temperature until it's just right.

Step into the shower and feel the water as it cascades over your shoulders and down your back.

Position your head so that water pours over your hair, neck, and face.

Pick up a bottle of shampoo and examine it. Notice its shape and design and how it feels in your hand.

Pour some shampoo into the palm of your hand. Notice its texture, color, and fragrance.

Massage the shampoo onto your hair. Feel the bubbly lather and the tingling of your scalp.

Rinse your hair and watch the bubbles swirl in a circle while approaching the drain.

Pick up a bar of soap and examine it visually. Notice its shape, color, texture, and fragrance.

Start washing your body. Notice the look and feel of the lather on your arms, hands, and fingers; and on your legs, feet, and toes.

Rinse your body and notice how the lather dissolves.

Position your face under the water. Close your eyes, open your mouth, and extend your tongue. Feel the droplets strike the surface of your tongue.

Allow a small amount of clear, clean water to enter your mouth. Then, close your mouth. Swirl the water around your tongue and mouth. Feel its liquid warmth. Swallow a small amount of water and follow the sensation as it passes your throat and gradually descends all the way down to your stomach.

Turn off the water and notice how the showerhead continues to drip, and listen to the last drops of water as they fall to the shower floor.

Reach for a towel. Notice its color and texture. Dry your body from head to toe. Notice the sensations of your warm, moist skin as it becomes dry. Notice how fresh and clean your body feels. Appreciate this feeling and offer a short, silent prayer of gratitude. Daily activities are pleasurable when you choose to be mindful.

★★★

A Morning Pledge

I've awakened to a day of hope and promise
Endless opportunities await me

I pledge to live fully in the present moment
And to look upon the world with compassionate eyes

Washing and Blessing of Hands

As water flows over my hands, may God bless them
May I use them carefully and skillfully
May I use them to comfort and heal

★★★

Meditation guidelines ...

Fundamentally, there are two types of meditation. The first one asks you to either focus on a stationary object, or repeat a chosen mantra. This method uses the power of concentration to keep your mind from producing thoughts. The second type of meditation asks you to focus on breathing in and breathing out. This insight-based technique suggests that your thoughts be calmly recognized, and then dismissed. It requires letting go of random thoughts before they are spun into a story and you grow attached to them. Again, withhold judgment on your thoughts – don't label them "good" or "bad."

★★★

Meditation is a spiritual journey that unfolds in a kind heart and quiet mind. Meditation helps you understand that thoughts and their attached emotions are often without merit. In truth, you needn't act on every thought that crosses your mind.

Choose a quiet place and a time when you won't be interrupted.

Determine ahead of time how long you want to meditate. Ten minutes is a good starting point, and you can set a timer if you wish.

Find a comfortable position. You can sit upright in a chair or on the floor. Or, you can recline or lie down. Realize that reclining or lying down may cause you to fall asleep, which is not your desired outcome.

Begin by gently closing your eyes and do a head to toe body scan. Soften any muscles that might be rigid or tense. Relax, no squeezing or clenching.

As you continue to focus on your body, make note of any physical sensations. Is there any pain or discomfort? Is your body weak or strong? Is your body tired or energized? Simply be aware of these sensations without judging them.

Next, focus on your breathing. Be fully aware of each breath that comes in, and each breath that goes out. This intense concentration on inhaling and exhaling will help your mind be free of thoughts. Notice how breathing in feels different from breathing out. Be aware of the subtle distinctions found in the beginning, middle, and end of each breath.

When you recognize that your attention has wandered – when you notice a thought or distraction – gently let go of that thought or distraction. Direct your focus back to the physical sensations of breathing in and out.

Don't be upset over your lapses in concentration. They are expected. It isn't a question of *if* you will stray, only *when* you will stray. All you need to do is start over, to redirect your full attention to the physical sensations of breathing in and breathing out.

When your mind is void of all thoughts, you have entered a holy space. This time is healing, and it will be your anchor, your rock. This time will be a peace-filled sanctuary in a turbulent world. It will be a safe and sacred destination you can visit over and over again.

With practice, you will become more proficient. Gradually lengthen your meditation time to twenty or thirty minutes, or perhaps longer. Because it strengthens your ability to live in the present moment, meditation allows you to celebrate life's joys; and it empowers you to face a crisis with greater clarity, calmness, and resolve.

★★★

In addition to the most common, thought-free meditation presented above, there are other kinds of meditational techniques. Try the following breathing exercises that are very easy, yet restorative.

Breathing Meditation #1

In-Breath: *I know that anger makes me ugly*
Out-Breath: *I don't want to be disfigured*
In-Breath: *I know that I must find harmony*
Out-Breath: *Forgiveness is the only answer*

Breathing Meditation #2

In–Breath: *Breathing in makes me calm*
Out–Breath: *Breathing out I release*
In–Breath: *Breathing in makes me smile*
Out–Breath: *Breathing out brings me peace*
In–Breath: *There is only this moment*
Out–Breath: *It is a wonderful moment*

Breathing Meditation #3

In–Breath: *My mind can go in a thousand directions*
Out–Breath: *But on this path, I walk in stillness*
In–Breath: *With each step, I am humbled by beauty*
Out–Breath: *With each step, I am closer to God*

Breathing Meditation #4

In–Breath: *I breathe in love*
Out–Breath: *I breathe out fear*
In–Breath: *I breathe in light*
Out–Breath: *I breathe out darkness*
In–Breath: *I breathe in what is happening*
Out–Breath: *I breathe out judgment*
In–Breath: *I breathe in acceptance*
Out–Breath: *I breathe out resistance*
In–Breath: *I breathe in healing*
Out–Breath: *I breathe out pain*

Inspired by Thich Nhat Hanh

★★★

In order to fall asleep, we need to stop thinking. In that sense, we need to learn how to fall asleep. Mindfulness, then, is learning how to "fall awake" by living in the present moment.

★★★

The past is just a memory, and the future is but a dream. Everything that's real and meaningful is unfolding now.

★★★

Evidence of God's presence is found not only in the extraordinary, but in the ordinary as well. You just have to search a bit harder.

★★★

Closing reflection ...

How might improved mindfulness skills make you a better caregiver? A better parent or partner? Is it worth an investment of your time and effort to gain these skills?

★★★

DAY THREE

ECKHART TOLLE

> There is a potentially redemptive dimension to
> every tragedy and disaster. *Eckhart Tolle*

★★★

Born in the Ruhr Valley of Germany, Eckhart Tolle endured a troubled and unhappy childhood. He struggled with fear and anxiety, a problem that would haunt him for many years. Tolle's parents divorced, and Eckhart, at age thirteen, chose to live with his father who was working in Spain. In his late teens, Tolle was tormented by severe bouts of depression. He moved again, this time to England, and managed to earn a degree from the University of London. But Tolle, now in his mid-twenties, dropped out of an elite postgraduate program at Cambridge University. He then spent several years drifting aimlessly and fighting suicidal impulses. Family members were alarmed. A few actually questioned his sanity, while others thought Tolle's behavior ranged somewhere between disturbingly irresponsible and frightfully bizarre.

As an avowed atheist, he often reflected on his own vulnerability and mortality. A persistent inner voice convinced Tolle that he was living a life of misery, a life that was trapped between a regretful past and a fearful future. Taking refuge inside the cramped room of a shabby boardinghouse, Tolle wondered how such a promising life had fallen apart. He thought, *I can't live with myself any longer.* Then, an intriguing question arose: Who is the "I" that can't live with the self? Haunted by this enigma, Tolle reclined on a tiny cot. He tossed and turned, finally drifting into a dream state. During this surreal time, he was cognizant of an observing awareness, a silent witness to his dreams.

After awakening, the same silent observer was still present. Tolle understood that, in truth, this primal awareness had *always* been there and would forever *be* there. And though it was part of him, he knew the awareness would outlive his body. He knew that the silent witness was not only real, it was invulnerable and immortal as well. And yet another breakthrough surfaced. Tolle realized that his own mind was responsible for crafting his make-believe world of suffering. His mind had shaped all of his negative, misguided perceptions. He had, in fact, allowed his undisciplined mind to arrogantly judge that life was unbearable and not worth living. Feeling as if a giant weight had been lifted from his shoulders, he thought, *I can **choose** to live with myself!* Tolle slept soundly for the first time in months, and he awoke to a profound and lasting inner peace.

For the next two years, Tolle spent much of his time sitting on a London park bench that overlooked an idyllic pond. He was happier than ever before. And while watching ducks frolic on the water, Tolle gained additional insights which served as material for his first book, *The Power of Now.* He began living a contemplative life, practicing meditation and studying the world's major religions. Tolle went on to write another bestseller titled, *A New Earth.* Combined, these two books have sold more than eight million copies and are available in thirty-three languages.

★★★

Eckhart Tolle: Thoughts and reflections ...

True freedom is living as if you had actually chosen whatever you feel or experience at this moment.

Had you not suffered, there would be no depth to you as a human being, no humility or compassion. Therefore, suffering is necessary until you realize it is unnecessary.

With stillness comes its benediction: peace.

Just as you're renewed by a respite from busyness, you are cleansed by a respite from thoughts.

Death is the most natural thing in the world, inseparable from its polarity: birth. Remind yourself of this when sitting with a dying person.

If there were only one color – blue, for instance – and the entire world and everything in it were blue, then there would be no blue.

Whenever a life form dies, God shines through the opening left by the dissolving form. That is why death is sacred; and that is why the peace of God can come to you through the acceptance of death.

By confronting death, your consciousness is freed, to some extent, from identification with form. That's why certain Buddhist traditions encourage monks to visit morgues and meditate among dead bodies.

Cultures that shun death inevitably become shallow and superficial, concerned only with the external form of things.

When death is denied, life loses its richness.

Pain cannot make you unhappy. Only your thoughts, judgments, and manufactured stories about pain can make you unhappy.

If you were nothing more than thoughts, then you wouldn't even know you are thinking. You would be like a dreamer who doesn't know he's dreaming.

Thoughts cannot exist without consciousness, but consciousness does not require thoughts.

Life gives you whatever is most helpful, including pain. How do you know what you need? You need whatever is happening now.

All the things that truly matter – beauty, love, creativity, joy, inner peace – transcend the mind and its thoughts.

The primary cause of unhappiness has nothing to do with an event or a situation; rather, it's your thoughts about it.

You must be able to distinguish thoughts from awareness and be able to separate them. You must realize that awareness is the space in which thoughts exist.

Your true self transcends all thinking. While your thoughts may be important, they do not define you.

★★★

Don't confuse content with context. Having little to do with *what* happens, **now** is the *space* in which things happen. As you become more completely immersed in **now**, you tend to have fewer thoughts – your mind becomes more quiet and still. Then, you start to realize that your true nature is much deeper than mere thoughts, and that **now** is more profound than any content which might arise. Thoughts, feelings, and experiences comprise life's content; and for most of us, life is good when the content is desirable – that is, when the pathway is smooth.

Another aspect of human nature is that people perceive themselves as only a body. This explains why someone's quality of life is typically tied to his or her health. But exciting changes are within reach as you adopt an expanded self-perception. In an interconnected universe, for example, are you not joined to the timelessness of **now**? And could it be that your human essence is, in part, the changeless space in which life unfolds? By virtue of these added insights, you may confidently proclaim: *I am more than my thoughts, my feelings, and my experiences. I am more than just a body.* At this point, life's content is secondary, and you're no longer a slave to time. And that means you're less likely to be disappointed or demoralized.

★★★

All that is essential is invisible to the eye.

★★★

Fear lurks within anger. The ego prefers anger over fear, believing that anger holds a higher moral standing.

★★★

Small obstacles and aggravations tend to accumulate. Then, some little thing goes wrong and there's an unexpected explosion of anger and frustration. It's an ego-driven frenzy – an overreaction that releases all of your suppressed feelings, not just the ones tied to the insignificant trigger event.

★★★

Closing reflection ...

Tolle's Four Steps to Success

1. Use obstacles as opportunities.
2. Separate your identity from your thinking.
3. Distance yourself from negativity.
4. Spend time in an environment that sparks creativity.

If you were to apply these principles at work and at home, how might your life be improved?

★★★

DAY FOUR

AWE THERAPY

> There's so much mystery, so much awe in the world
> that science can't explain. *Jane Goodall*

★★★

Have you ever been awestruck? By definition, awe is witnessing or feeling the presence of something vast and beyond human scale. It's experiencing something that transcends the common and mundane, something that challenges our current understanding of the world. Perhaps you've felt awe while gazing at the Milky Way, visiting Niagara

Falls, or climbing a mountain. Yet simple, humble moments can also inspire awe, such as when a baby looks at you and smiles.

So it may not be surprising that awe has captured the attention of researchers. A three-year project, funded by the Templeton Foundation and run by the University of California, sheds new light on the mystery of awe. For a long time, only the primary emotions – happiness, sadness, fear, anger, disgust, and surprise – were deemed worthy of scientific interest. But groundbreaking studies have revealed four important aspects to awe.

First, awe brings people together. In other words, when viewing a grand vista or a starry sky, we realize that we're a small part of something much larger. This realization urges us to work more collaboratively with people, and to be more helpful. Suddenly, we're thinking less about ourselves and more about others.

Secondly, awe enhances mindfulness and, therefore, helps us be calm and attentive. In addition, mindfulness prepares us to be more receptive and responsive to whatever challenges might come our way. Perhaps that's why Albert Einstein identified awe as the source of all true art and science.

Next, awe makes us nicer. It inspires people to act more kindly, generously, and ethically. An innovative experiment demonstrated this point. Volunteers were divided into two groups, with each group looking at a picture for sixty seconds. The first group gazed at a picture of eucalyptus trees, while the second group viewed a nondescript building. Of course, the tree-gazers reported greater awe. And when the test leader "accidentally" dropped pencils that scattered on the floor, the awestruck people responded much faster and picked up more pencils than the other test group.

And fourth, awe changes our bodies and minds. As we experience awe, the body's level of cytokines, an inflammation marker linked to depression, is significantly reduced. Experts have also proven that awe therapy – in essence, exposure to nature's beauty – lowers blood pressure, slows pulse rates, and strengthens immune systems.

★★★

Meet Stacy Bare, an army veteran who suffered from PTSD following his second deployment to Iraq. He was drinking heavily, withdrawing from his family, and struggling with suicidal thoughts. Bare's counselor suggested hiking and rock climbing as part of his therapy. Did a pinch of awe and a dose of exercise prove helpful? Bare thinks so, as evidenced by him saying, "I literally climbed out of depression."

★★★

For thousands of years, early humans were deeply connected to the world around them; for their very survival was tied to finding food, water, and shelter. Their intimate connection with nature included expressions of gratitude for water, rocks, and soil; and for fish, birds, animals, plants, and trees. Their thanksgiving extended to the sun, the rain, the moon, the stars, the tides, the seasons – and yes, the beauty and wonder of it all. These ancient people recognized and celebrated awe, even as they were immersed in it. They lived in caves, adobe houses, grass huts, and frame shelters covered by animal hides. They walked the deserts, forests, and mountain ranges. In primitive boats, they explored lakes, rivers, and seas. Our attraction to nature is undeniable. We're intuitively drawn to beauty, because we yearn for healing. And we instinctively search for awe, because goodness is in our DNA.

★★★

Finding awe in everyday life ...

Take time to gaze at the clouds or stars.
Make a point to watch a sunrise or sunset.
Reflect on a time in your life when you experienced awe.
Visit a museum or planetarium.
Explore a local, state, or national park.

Take a walk, seeing everything as if it were the first time.
Observe children interacting on a playground or in a pool.
Watch a game of pick-up basketball.
Check out an amazing cathedral.
Attend a live concert.

★★★

It's rare to be outdoors in a place so remote that you can't hear man-made sounds: no droning televisions or radios; no lawnmowers or motorcycles; no distant cars or trucks, trains or planes. Most likely, something will catch your ear: a buzzing bee, a moaning tree, a chirping bird. Or perhaps there will be complete silence. If you find such a place, pause and cherish the moment; for you've come upon a heaven-like sanctuary.

★★★

Is it not possible for any space to be holy, for any place to be a sanctuary of peace or an altar of praise? Once your mind perceives a place as sacred, your heart will take over and make it so.

★★★

Signs of abundance can trigger awe – spectacles like golden fields of grain stretching beyond the horizon, a background of majestic, snow-capped mountains, or the dazzling brilliance of a sun-drenched, afternoon sky. And have you noticed the noble splendor exhibited by large herds of animals? Or have you marveled at the mindful grace displayed by huge flocks of migrating birds? Still, organic life and nature's beauty aren't the only sources of awe and wonder. Fueled by our creative instincts, men and women have designed and constructed elegant buildings that penetrate the clouds, and we've engineered and built breathtaking bridges that link the accessible to the unreachable.

★★★

Spiritual teachers suggest that, in order to bring heaven to earth, you must see the world through childlike eyes. That is to say, you should strive to view the world through a lens of innocence and wonder. Of course, childlike awe has nothing to do with childishness, and has little in common with petulant, childish behavior.

★★★

Today, I am in awe of the one Spirit
And the diverse creations born of the one Spirit

Today, everything and everyone belong
And I forgive what I cannot understand

Today, I teach love and compassion
Kindness and helpfulness

Today, my childlike eyes see only innocence and perfection
Beauty and abundance

Today, I feel an infinite Divine presence
As I choose to follow my heart

Immersed in this moment, I am humble and grateful
Jubilant and triumphant!

★★★

Studies have shown that looking at a picture of a forest reduces stress; and reading a soothing poem reduces stress as well. What's more, research indicates that looking thoughtfully at religious icons will elevate your consciousness, and listening to the choral music of Beethoven will do the same. Here's the point. It *does* matter what you choose to watch, listen to, and read. In fact, these choices significantly impact your life. Wellness includes recognizing and appreciating what is true, beautiful, and holy. And a critical element of intentionality is to purposefully connect with truth, beauty, and holiness – knowing that it promotes well-being and inner peace.

★★★

Breathe deeply and celebrate this moment
Do this and find peace
Dare to experience wholeness

Be immersed in what is true, beautiful, and holy
Do this and begin to heal
Dare to be born again!

★★★

Philosophy was born the moment humans first gazed at the night sky and experienced a deep sense of awe and wonder. Soon thereafter, questions arose – questions that ultimately led to extraordinary advances in both physics and metaphysics. By definition, philosophy explores the fundamental nature of knowledge, reality, and existence. It is, therefore, a dynamic discipline that mirrors the fluid, ever-changing fabric of life. Philosophies are usually a mix of scientific evidence and religious or spiritual beliefs. This blend of information creates a foundational point of reference that shapes our perceptions of the world and everything we experience. This fixed point of reference – our core values and principles – helps us cope with episodes of upheaval and tragedy. Only a profound awakening will cause someone to change the current, familiar lens through which he or she views the world.

★★★

In his philosophy of the good, the true, and the beautiful, Plato offered the following insights:

Good: Morals, Culture, Ethics

True: Science, Nature, Logic

Beautiful: Art, Self, Aesthetics

A parallel philosophy – the good, the true, the beautiful, and the holy – offers these guidelines:

Good: Kindness, Charity, Humility

True: Life, Knowledge, Awareness

Beautiful: Spirit, Love, Creativity

Holy: Divinity, Covenants, Sacraments

What commonalities do the two philosophies share? What are the biggest differences between them? Which philosophy do you find more appealing? Why?

★★★

A Hymn of Praise

For the beauty of the earth,
For the glory of the skies,
For the love which from our birth
Over and around us lies;
Lord of all to thee we raise
This our hymn of grateful praise.

For the beauty of each hour
Of the day and of the night,
Hill and vale and tree and flower,
Sun and moon and stars of light;
Lord of all to thee we raise
This our hymn of grateful praise.

For the joy of ear and eye,
For the heart and mind's delight,

For the mystic harmony
Linking sense to sound and sight;
Lord of all to thee we raise
This our hymn of grateful praise.

By Folliott Sanders Pierpoint

★★★

Closing reflection ...

Albert Einstein suggested there are two ways to perceive the world: Everything is a miracle, or nothing is a miracle. If you were to choose, from this moment forward, to see everything as a miracle, how might that outlook change your life?

For you, what things inspire awe? Try to describe the feeling of awe. How does awe impact your body? How does awe affect your mind? Your spirit?

Can you recall any care giving experiences that triggered awe? If so, how do these occasions affect the way you feel about your hospice work?

★★★

DAY FIVE

POETRY

Poetry is an echo, asking a shadow to dance. *Carl Sandberg*

★★★

An elegant cluster of words – with or without rhyme and cadence – is a beautiful thing. Not only does poetry offer contemplative opportunities, it has the power to lift your spirit and lighten your heart. Poetry holds the potential to inform and inspire, to comfort and soothe. A thoughtful verse artfully crafted transcends culture and ideology. By all measures, the ageless poems of Rumi and Hafiz have reached this lofty summit. Revered by critics, scholars, and casual readers alike, their collective works are known for exuberant expressions of love and joy, accompanied by splashes of humor and whimsy.

Rumi was born in the Middle East at the beginning of the 13th century, and Hafiz, who studied and admired Rumi's poetry, was born in the same region during the 14th century. Both were Sufi masters, men who were transformed by direct, personal experiences with God. And clearly, their insights and views of the human experience are timeless.

With this brief history as a backdrop, find a quiet place to read and enjoy the following selection of poems. Then, reflect on their humble, yet sublime lessons. You'll find that each poem is graced by layered meaning. So if you're willing to peel the onion, hidden slivers of Divinity may be revealed.

★★★

Don't run around this world
looking for a hole to hide in.

There are wild beasts in every cave!
If you live with mice,
the cat claws will find you.

The only rest comes
when you're alone with God.

Live in the nowhere that you came from,
even though you have an address here.

You have eyes that see from that nowhere,
and eyes that judge distances,
how high and how low.

You own two shops,
and you run back and forth.

Keep open the shop
where you're not selling fishhooks anymore.
You *are* the free-swimming fish.

Rumi

★★★

Someone who goes with half a loaf of bread
to a small place that fits like a nest around him,
someone who wants no more,
who's not himself longed for by anyone else,
he is a letter to everyone.

You open it.
It says, *Live!*

Rumi

★★★

The mystery does not get clearer by repeating the question,
nor is it bought by going to amazing places.

Until you've kept your eyes
and your wanting still for fifty years,
you don't begin to cross over from confusion.

Rumi

★★★

The same wind that uproots trees
makes the grasses shine.

The lordly wind loves the weakness
and the lowness of grasses.
Never brag of being strong.

Does a flame consider the size of the woodpile?
The axe doesn't worry how thick the branches are.
It cuts them to pieces. But not the leaves.
It leaves the leaves alone.

What is form in the presence of reality?
Reality keeps the sky turned over
like a cup above us, revolving.
Who turns the sky wheel?

And the motion of the body comes
from the spirit like a waterwheel
that's held in a stream.

The inhaling-exhaling is from the spirit,
now angry, now peaceful.
Wind destroys, and wind protects.
This never ends.

Rumi

★★★

Solomon was busy judging others,
when it was his personal thoughts
which were disrupting the community.

His crown slid crooked on his head.
He put it straight, but the crown went
awry again. Eight times this happened.

Finally he began to talk to his headpiece.
"Why do you keep tilting over my eyes?"

"I have to. When your power loses compassion,
I have to show what such a condition looks like."

Immediately Solomon recognized the truth.
He knelt and asked forgiveness.
The crown centered itself on his crown.

When something goes wrong,
accuse yourself first. Wisdom can wobble
and go blind.

Listen when your crown reminds you
of what makes you cold toward others,
as you pamper the greedy thoughts inside.

Rumi

★★★

The breeze at dawn has secrets to tell you.
Don't go back to sleep.

You must ask for what you really want.
Don't go back to sleep.

People are going back and forth across the door sill
where the two worlds touch.

The door is round and open.
Don't go back to sleep.

Rumi

★★★

Out beyond the ideas of right-doing and wrong-doing,
there is a field. I'll meet you there.

When the soul lies down in that grass,
the world is too full to talk about.
Ideas, language, even the phrase *each other*
doesn't make any sense.

Rumi

★★★

Inside this new love, die.
Your way begins on the other side.
Become the sky.
Take an axe to the prison wall.
Escape.
Walk out like someone suddenly born into color.
Do it now.
You're covered by a thick cloud.
Slide out the side. Die,
and be quiet. Quietness is the surest sign
that you've died.
Your old life was a frantic running from silence.

The speechless full moon
comes out now.

Rumi

★★★

Do you think I know what I'm doing?
That for one breath or half-breath I belong to myself?
As much as a pen knows what it's writing,
or the ball can guess where it's going next.

Rumi

★★★

Late, by myself, in the boat of myself,
no light and no land anywhere,
cloud cover thick. I try to stay
just above the surface, yet I'm already under
and living within the ocean.

Rumi

★★★

This being human is a guest house.
Every morning a new arrival.

A joy, a depression, a meanness,
some momentary awareness comes
as an unexpected visitor.

Welcome and entertain them all!
Even if they're a crowd of sorrows,
who violently sweep your house
empty of its furniture,
still, treat each guest honorably.
He may be clearing you out
for some new delight.

The dark thought, the shame, the malice,
meet them at the door laughing,
and invite them in.

Be grateful for whoever comes,
because each has been sent
as a guide from beyond.

Rumi

★★★

Does sunset sometimes look like the sun's coming up?

John A. Love

Do you know what a faithful love is like?

You're crying. You say you've burned yourself.
But can you think of anyone who's not
·hazy with smoke?

Rumi

★★★

What is the root of all these words?
One thing: love.

But a love so deep and sweet
It needed to express itself
With scents, sounds, colors
That never before existed.

Hafiz

★★★

Every child has known God,
Not the God of names,
Not the God of don'ts,
Not the God who does something scary,
But the God who only knows four words
And keeps repeating them, saying:
"Come dance with me."
Come
Dance.

Hafiz

★★★

Once a man came to me and spoke for hours about
His great vision of God.

He asked, "Are these wondrous dreams true?"

I replied, "How many goats do you have?"

He looked surprised and said,
"I'm speaking of Divine visions
And you ask about goats!"

And I spoke again saying,
"Yes, brother – how many do you have?"

"Well, I have sixty-two."

Then I said,
"You asked me if your God dreams are true,
I would say that they are if they make you become
More human, more loving,
More kind to every creature that you know."

Hafiz

★★★

I am a hole in a flute
That the Christ-breath moves through.
Listen to this music.

I am the concert
From the mouth of every creature
Singing with the myriad chords.

Hafiz

★★★

It is not easy to stop
Thinking ill of others.

Usually one must enter
Into a friendship with a person
Who has accomplished that
Great feat himself.

Then something might start to
Rub off on you
Of that true elegance.

Hafiz

★★★

All of your images of winter
I see against your sky.

I understand the wounds
That have not healed in you.

They exist because God and love
Have yet to become real enough
To let you forgive the dream.

Hafiz

★★★

Greatness
Is always built upon this foundation:
The ability
To appear, speak, and act
As the most
Common
Man.

Hafiz

★★★

God
Blooms
From the shoulder
Of the
Elephant
Who becomes
Courteous
To the
Ant.

Hafiz

★★★

If this world were not held in God's bucket
How could an ocean stand upside down
On its head and never lose a drop?

If your life were not contained in God's cup
How could you be so brave and laugh
And dance in the face of death?

God has written a thousand promises
All over your heart,
Your life has been sealed and marked
"Too sacred, too sacred to ever end!"

Hafiz

★★★

You carry all the ingredients
To turn your life into a nightmare,
Don't mix them!

You have all the genius
To build a swing in your backyard
For God.

That sounds like a lot more fun.
Start laughing, planning
And gathering friends.

You carry all the ingredients
To live a life of joy,
Mix them, mix them!

Hafiz

★★★

No
One
In need of love
Can sit with my verse for
An hour
And then walk away without carrying
Golden tools,
And feeling that God
Just came
Near.

Hafiz

★★★

Why just ask the donkey in me
To speak to the donkey in you,

When I have so many other beautiful animals
And brilliantly colored birds inside
That are longing to say something wonderful
And exciting to your heart?

Hafiz

★★★

Now is the time to know
That everything you do is sacred.

Now is the time to know
That your every thought is holy.

Now is the season to know
That there is nothing but grace.

Now is the season to make
A lasting truce with God.

Hafiz

★★★

Closing reflection ...

It's ironic that such gentle, tender poetry was penned in one of the most troubled regions of the world – a part of the world that, to this day, is ruled by theocratic and autocratic nations mired in war and violence. How are beautiful poems created in the midst of pain and suffering? What does this say about human nature?

Even in the world's darkest places, points of light emerge. They are beacons of hope that serve as guides for the lost.

When you read a poem that touches your heart, you are connecting with the writer on a deep, human level. The poet's age, gender, and race are irrelevant; and religious and political views are of no importance, for humanity's endowments extend far beyond such distinctions.

★★★

DAY SIX

MANAGING ANXIETY

> To enjoy good health and bring peace to all, you
> must discipline and control your mind. *Buddha*

★★★

Statistics indicate that, in the United States alone, roughly 40 million men, women, and children are struggling with an anxiety disorder. In fact, there's a one in three chance that you *will* have a panic attack at some point in your life. Anxiety types fall into three major groups: generalized anxiety, social anxiety, and panic disorder. Here's a quick overview of these three types of anxiety and their associated symptoms.

Panic disorder is marked by fear that's linked to the possibility of having a panic attack. Symptoms include rapid heart rate, hyperventilation, dizziness, and nausea. Generalized anxiety is marked by excessive worry about normal, everyday things that are part of life. It typically includes a deep and lasting sense of dread or doom which stands in the way of more desirable feelings like contentment, happiness, and joy. Finally, social anxiety is marked by an avoidance of settings and activities that trigger physical responses such as blushing, trembling, or sweating – which, in turn, lead to fear of embarrassment.

Have you experienced any of these feelings? If so, how often? If you have frequent or severe episodes of anxiety, consider seeking professional help. Sometimes, medicine is appropriate for managing symptoms. But either way, a licensed therapist can guide you through the interventions needed to allay your fear and improve your quality of life.

Each of the three types of anxiety has physical, mental, and behavioral symptoms. In other words, to effectively manage anxiety, you must soothe your anxious body, calm your anxious mind, and tame your anxious behavior. Fortunately, there are proven, self-help techniques available, such as those suggested by anxiety management expert, Dr. Margaret Wehrenberg. Because her methods promote calmness, they help nearly everyone. So if nerves have ever made you feel like a butterfly was in your stomach, or a rock was in your gut, there's good news. These unpleasant sensations are not only common, they're relatively easy to manage. Let's examine some of the powerful interventions that Wehrenberg and other respected therapists recommend.

To soothe your anxious body, try breathing from your diaphragm.

Unlike the shallow breaths that come from your chest, deep breaths supported by your diaphragm promote healthy physiological changes almost instantly. Deep breathing techniques have proven to be, in fact, the most reliable way to prevent a panic attack, and the best way to stop an attack once it has begun. So how can you know if you're breathing from the diaphragm? Start by placing your hand over the lower part of the stomach as you breathe in and out. If your hand remains stationary, then you are breathing from your chest. If, however, your hand moves outward as you inhale, and it moves inward as you exhale, then you're breathing properly, with support coming from the diaphragm. You must practice this deep, diaphragm-strengthened breathing – and become proficient – before moving on to more advanced techniques.

While working on your deep breathing skills, remember to focus wholly on each in-breath and each out-breath. By closing your eyes, you're less likely to be distracted. Breathe slowly and mindfully; and as your concentration improves, fewer random thoughts will cross your mind. When a thought does creep in, simply dismiss it. The long-term goal is for your mind to be a blank slate: quiet and absent of thoughts. Though deep breathing is simple, it isn't easy. But as deep breathing becomes more natural, you won't forget how to do it when a fearful situation arises and anxiety knocks at the door.

Here's an effective, yet easy, ten-step breathing exercise.

1. Inhale to the count of two
2. Exhale to the count of two
3. Inhale to the count of two
4. Exhale to the count of four
5. Inhale to the count of two
6. Exhale to the count of six
7. Inhale to the count of two
8. Exhale to the count of eight
9. Inhale to the count of two
10. Exhale to the count of ten

To soothe your anxious body, try relaxing your muscles.

Muscle tightness is often caused by mental tension. So if you've already experienced a panic attack, you might worry about having another one – and that worry will lead to muscle tightness. If you have social anxiety, muscle tightness will occur prior to a public outing. Or if you have generalized anxiety, your mind is frequently on high alert – and that, too, will produce muscle tightness.

Progressive muscle relaxation is the preferred treatment to release tightness. The goal is to relax all of your muscle groups in a single, structured exercise. The following muscle relaxation technique takes about ten minutes to complete. However, committed practice can cut that time in half.

- Start by sitting upright.
- Close your eyes and begin your diaphragm-supported, deep breathing.
- Focus on the sensations of each muscle group
- Gently drop your head forward with your chin tucked to your chest; hold, and then return your head to its upright position. Now, slowly lean your head backward; hold, and then return your head to its upright position. Gently tilt your head to the left side; hold, and return your head to its upright position. Now,

slowly tilt your head to the right side; hold, and return your head to its upright position. Notice the release of tension. Feel the warmth and the renewed energy. Repeat x 3.

- Moving to your scalp, raise your eyebrows to tighten the scalp; hold, then release. Repeat x 3

- Moving to your forehead, furrow your brow to tighten the skin; hold, then release. Repeat x 3

- Now, squint your eyes, wrinkle your nose, and purse your lips; hold, then release. Repeat x 3

- Next, move to your shoulders. Raise them up; hold, then release. Repeat x 3

- Now, to your arms. Clench your left fist to tighten your forearm, wrist, hand and fingers; hold, then release. Do exactly the same by clenching your right fist; hold, then release. Repeat x 3

- Next, move to your back and abdomen. Tighten this area by imagining a string pulling your belly button towards your spine; hold, then release. Repeat x 3

- Now, to your buttocks. Tighten by squeezing together; hold, then release. Repeat x 3

- Next, move to your thighs. Tighten your left quad muscles; hold, then release. Do exactly the same by tightening your right quad muscles; hold, then release. Repeat x 3

- Now, to your calves and shins. Tighten by pointing the toes of your left foot downward. Feel the shin muscles stretch and the calf muscles contract; hold, then release. Do exactly the same by pointing the toes of your right foot downward; hold, then release. Repeat x 3

- Next, move to your feet. Curl the toes of your left foot and press your left heal to the floor; hold, then release. Do exactly the same by curling the toes of your right foot and pressing your right heel to the floor; hold, then release. Repeat x 3

- Notice how you feel so relaxed, warm, and peaceful. Your body says, "Thank you!"

To soothe your anxious body, try shifting your awareness.

By its nature, anxiety is founded on either what has happened in the past or what might happen in the future. The present moment, therefore, is the best friend of those who are troubled by anxiety. If something frightening is happening at this very instant, you're probably just dealing with it — there isn't time for you to be worried or anxious. Simply stated, you are safe in this present moment. That's why mindfulness has a calming effect. What's more, a calm state allows you to think more clearly and find an optimal solution to whatever problem arises.

Yet, there's another key advantage to mindfulness. Within the boundary of living in the present moment, you can focus either inward or outward. The choice is yours, and here's why it matters. If something "out there" is scary, you can turn inward. Conversely, if something "inside" is ominous, you can focus outward. It's called shifting your awareness, and you gain a sense of control because *you* decide which direction to turn. If, for example, you are fearful of sweating and you focus on that possible outcome, then you will inevitably start to sweat. But in that same scenario, if you turn your awareness to the world around you — to anything, be it sublime or mundane — that dreaded sweating episode your mind envisioned won't actually happen.

The following exercise allows you to practice this technique, and make it a valuable asset to your toolbox.

1. Close your eyes. Now, slowly inhale through your nose. Direct your full awareness on this deep inward breath. Notice every aspect of it: your flaring nostrils; the coolness of the air as it passes through your throat; your expanding lungs; your shifting clothes ...
2. Now, slowly exhale through your nose. Direct your full awareness to this outward airflow. Notice every aspect of it: the warmth of the air as it passes through your throat; your shrinking lungs; your shifting clothes ...

3. With eyes still closed, slowly inhale through your nose. Direct your full awareness to the world around you. Notice every aspect of it: every sound; every smell; every movement …

4. Open your eyes. Now, slowly exhale through your nose. Direct your full awareness to the world around you. Notice every aspect of what you see: every object; every person; every activity … Repeat this four-step sequence x 3

To calm your anxious mind, try redefining your catastrophes.

Sometimes your mind will perceive a given situation as truly awful or terrible. Next, you assume the worst is about to happen. It might start out with a panicked thought such as *Oh, no!* and quickly build from there. Soon, it becomes a full-blown catastrophe. Yet honestly, panic is just a feeling. It's unpleasant, but not lethal. Remind yourself of this, and then practice your deep breathing technique.

Dread and fear are also feelings you might experience, even when there aren't any actual threats. Remember this, and then focus your awareness away from whatever is triggering your dread or fear. The same holds true for embarrassment. It's just a feeling that cannot harm you. Shift your awareness and remind yourself that being noticed doesn't mean you're being rejected.

A thought like *I'm losing my mind!* is just an exaggerated myth, a destructive lie. In fact, worst case scenarios rarely happen. Remind yourself of this, and then focus on diaphragm-supported breathing. Recognizing and redefining your "catastrophes" will take you a long way towards calming your anxious mind.

To calm your anxious mind, try stopping your anxious thoughts.

It's normal to have anxious or negative thoughts from time to time. But when they become persistent, and perhaps relentless, you need to take action. Part of living in the present moment is monitoring your thoughts: Are they true? Are they helpful? Are they negative? Are they destructive? This kind of monitoring or "thought awareness" is a crucial responsibility that, of course, only you can manage. One of the most effective techniques to vanquish unwanted thoughts has two components: thought stopping and thought replacement.

When you first realize that you're stuck in a cycle of anxious or negative thoughts, say out loud: "Stop it!" Then, replace those disheartening thoughts by substituting positive, uplifting ones. Try reciting a poem or offering a prayer. Or you could sing a happy song, or redirect your mind by listening to music, playing a game, or reading a book. And finally, you might choose to focus on an enjoyable task, project, or hobby. Any one of these choices is much more rewarding and productive than hosting a pity party for yourself.

To calm your anxious mind, try containing your worries.

There are times when you just need to let go of everything on your mind, to sweep out the old and make way for the new. Here's an idea. Find a piece of paper and write down everything that's on your mind. Your list should be comprehensive, but make each entry very brief – this isn't a journaling exercise. When you're finished writing, place your list in a small box. Now, hold the box close to your heart, and offer a simple prayer, something like: Dear God, I give you my troubles and worries. I offer you all of my anxiety and fear. I trust you, and ask that you watch over me and keep me safe. Please help me feel your presence and your peace. Amen

To tame your anxious behavior, try managing your activities and achieving balance.

People with anxiety issues frequently compound their problems in one of two ways: Either they engage in too many activities, or else they're involved in activities that aren't rewarding. Sometimes, people take on too many duties because it's hard to say "no." But other times, they choose to stay overly busy because "free time" sparks anxiety.

If you happen to dread the times when there's nothing to do, consider this idea.

- Make a written list of things you would like to do if there were enough time. You can include any kind of activity, such as taking a bath, planting a garden, reorganizing the garage, rearranging your furniture, watching your favorite movie, and so on.
- Next, after each activity, write down the amount of time you might need to do it. It will be an estimated time, of course, but you should strive to have several activities that fall into structured time categories like thirty minutes, one hour, three hours, or an entire day.
- Carry this list with you, and whenever some unscheduled time comes up, choose something from your list that fits the available time. It will always be something you want to do, and it will relieve any mounting anxiety. As you complete an activity or task, cross it off and add a new one to the list.

If you happen to be a person who's trying to juggle too many balls, ask this question: Are your activities in harmony with your values? But before answering this query, take the time to analyze how you're currently spending time. Based on a typical workday, make a list of what you do – from the time you get up in the morning, until the time you go to bed – and how much time you spend on each activity. For example, if your day usually starts at 7:00AM and ends around 11:00PM, then you have sixteen hours to account for. Repeat the process, this time basing it on a nonworking day. Next, by combining the two lists and by factoring in your number of working days versus non-working days in a seven day week, you'll have a pretty clear picture of how you spend your time. You're off to a great start, but there's still more to do.

Take time to examine your values. What's important to you? Advancing your career? Buying a house? Spending more time with loved ones? What things make your life worth living? Write down your values and prioritize them. Most people strive to maintain a degree of work–life balance. Let's say, for instance, that your prioritized list of values includes: family, work, exercise, hobbies, spiritual growth, social events, volunteering, and time alone. The last question is: In an ideal world, how many hours per week would you like to spend with family, work, exercise, hobbies, spiritual growth, social events, volunteering, and time alone? Once this is determined, all that remains is to compare how you spend your time *now* with how you *want* to spend your time.

The current way you spend your time is a reflection of the choices you make. But are these choices supporting the way you *want* to spend your time? Are there changes you can make to mitigate any existing conflicts? Are there changes you can make to achieve a more balanced life? These key questions are worth exploring. But a good place to start is learning to say "no" to new activities and added duties that take you even further away from your ideal world.

Bonus Tip: If you have a number of tasks to complete, it's likely that some will be more daunting or unpleasant than others. Do the most difficult job first, followed by the second hardest task … until you finish.

To tame your anxious behavior, try setting clear goals and building new skills.

Any proactive endeavor that builds more competence and confidence will also help ease your anxiety symptoms. And perhaps the best way to become more competent and confident is to strengthen your knowledge and skill. The first step of your journey is to set a goal:

Identify something you want to achieve, and be specific. For example, you could set a goal to lose ten pounds, or knit a sweater, or speak in public, or be a volunteer.

The second step is to determine whatever might prompt anxiety as you work to achieve your goal. So if your objective is to speak in public, you might be worried about sweating, blushing, or trembling. You've already learned some effective coping skills for these symptoms: deep breathing exercises and shifting awareness techniques. But you can expand your toolbox even more by reading books, attending workshops, and so on.

The third step is to break down your preparation – your skill building – into manageable steps, and work on them one by one. Taking "baby steps" keeps you moving forward without feeling overwhelmed.

Finally, practice in private. Again, using the example of public speaking, you might consider rehearsing in front of a mirror. After that, you could try speaking in front of one trusted friend. These are just a few practical suggestions which will help you gain confidence, build competence, and achieve your goals. By integrating these ideas, you'll be well on your way to taming anxious behavior.

MANAGING DEPRESSION

In the United States, about ten percent of men and twenty-five percent of women will, at some point in their life, experience depression. In fact, major depressive disorder is the leading cause of disability for Americans who are sixteen to forty-four years of age. And these numbers don't include the millions of people suffering from low-grade depression, such as persistent negativity. Yet, the effects of depression stretch far beyond quality of life issues. Employers, for example, absorb the costs of absenteeism and diminished productivity; and in America, treatment costs – typically covered by health insurance – are approaching thirty billion dollars per year.

Therapists and physicians have identified three hallmarks associated with depression. The first one is *depressed energy*. People with depression lack both physical and mental energy. They can't find the strength, or the will, to do activities which energize most people – things like taking a walk or riding a bike. The second hallmark is *depressed behavior.* People with depression often delve into compulsive tasks and routines which, in turn, leads to complete exhaustion. Additionally, they tend to isolate themselves from others. And the third hallmark is *depressed thinking.* That is, depressed people show signs of persistent rumination and negativity. Their hopeless and helpless thinking may even lead to self-inflicted injuries.

As with anxiety, the symptoms of depression can be anywhere from mild to severe. What's more, it's important to remember that periods of sadness are entirely normal. Such times are part of life and are endured by everyone. But if you have an episode of sadness or negativity that lasts six months or longer, please get help from a therapist or physician. In some cases, a prescribed drug is needed to balance the brain's chemistry. Other times, drug-free interventions work very well. And yes, there are self-help techniques you may wish to consider. Once again, because self-help methods enrich the day-to-day human experience, they are useful for nearly everyone. So if you're like most people – working through occasional cycles of mild depression or negativity – try these time-tested insights.

1. Appreciate yourself

Feelings of inadequacy and worthlessness are central to depressed thinking. These negative feelings deplete the energy you need to try new things, to rise up to a challenge, and to overcome lethargy. As a result, life becomes a vicious circle. Every task seems overwhelming. Every problem appears to be insurmountable. And each time you fail to complete a task or solve a problem, your feelings of inadequacy and worthlessness are reinforced. Your goal is to break this chain of negativity, and here's a good way to begin: Stop saying bad things about yourself! This includes the silent thoughts crossing your mind *and* the things you say about yourself to others.

Next, start focusing on your strengths and attributes. Make a written list of what you like about yourself, and be sure to examine your character. For instance, I am: kind, courageous, generous, compassionate, intelligent, considerate, polite, easy-going, dependable, honest, loyal, and forgiving. Carry this list with you, and read it several times each day. As you go down the list, you'll be reminded that, regardless of your negative thoughts, these attributes describe you!

Finally, stop comparing yourself to others. In truth, life is much more than a contest. There will always be someone with a bigger house, a newer car, thicker hair, and fewer wrinkles. Accept where you are right now. Then set goals that are meaningful to you, along with reasonable timelines for what you hope to accomplish.

2. Choose a buddy

Burnout is a chronic state of physical, emotional, and cognitive exhaustion induced by ongoing stress, especially work related stress. Because chronic stress is debilitating at every level, burnout is a predictor of heart disease, type II diabetes, hypertension, immune deficiencies, and cognitive decline. Early signs include: a lasting sense of depletion; fatigue that continues even after a good night's sleep; energy that isn't restored after several days of rest; and a tendency to get sick following a period of stress.

As time goes on, people with burnout become more compulsive about finishing their work. They may start neglecting personal care and hygiene. They are more likely to overeat, drink excessively, or abuse drugs. And they become isolated – losing interest in things that once gave them pleasure. Do any of these behaviors sound familiar? And as if this weren't enough, the more burned out you are, the less likely you are to recognize your problem. That's why it's essential to recruit a buddy, someone who will help you recognize your symptoms; guide you through your chosen healing interventions; and assess your progress.

The next question: Is there someone you can turn to? Ideally, it should be someone you can trust as an advocate. However, your buddy must also hold you accountable. People often turn to a respected colleague for this kind of help.

3. Recognize the goodness in others

Although you can't control what other people do, you *can* control what you pay attention to. Looking for goodness in others requires a purposeful decision to replace a negative filter with a positive one. It's an effective way to reverse a critical, judgmental trend. Because if you only see the faults in people, why would you want to be around them? And when you're willing to take the next step forward, you can offer a verbal comment on the attributes you observe in others. You may be surprised at how their faces light up. Moreover, your positive words will cause others to react more pleasantly to you, thereby enhancing your self-esteem. Kindness is a gift that keeps on giving.

4. Remember past joys

Take a moment to recall an event or an experience that was very enjoyable. Next, spend a few minutes remembering all of the details of this wonderful time in your life. Then, express your gratitude for the people or the special circumstances which were central to this joyful experience. Now, ask yourself a question: How can I repeat this kind of moment again? Perhaps you can only repeat a certain portion of it. But either way, make a firm commitment to repeat as much of the experience as you can, and do it sooner rather than later.

5. Do something that restores you

People who are depressed usually stop doing what is good for them. So not only is their brain chemistry unbalanced, their life is unbalanced as well. They've chosen to stop doing the things that restore them.

If you fall into this category, here's an idea. First, make a written list of restorative activities. Your list could include intellectual, artistic, or spiritual events – such as going to a lecture, a play, a concert, or a worship service. Or you could visit a zoo, sit by a lake, or take a walk in the woods. You could choose to play golf or tennis. You could go bowling or dancing. Your list might include creative endeavors such as knitting, painting a picture, baking, or arranging flowers. It could be a social outing, like meeting a friend for coffee. Or you could watch a favorite movie or take a relaxing bath. You get to choose the things on your list.

Now, pick three activities from your list. Mark them on your calendar – one new activity for each of the next three weeks – and do them! It can be fun and easy to add restorative balance to your life.

6. Remember that a feeling is just a feeling

Your mind is closely tied to your body. As a result, a bodily event will often prompt your mind to attach a feeling to it. If your face is flushed, you're feeling embarrassed. If your chest is flooded with warmth, you're feeling compassion. Yet, as soon as a feeling is identified and labeled, it starts to fade.

In a depressed state, your mind will label nearly every feeling or sensation as a negative one. In order to interrupt these predisposed responses – these automatic feelings of despair – it's necessary to slow down the labeling stage. Additionally, you need to identify a feeling and choose to *not* be alarmed by it. And it helps to remember that feelings, while they are real, do not always reflect truth or reality.

Sometimes, feelings of gloom and doom are triggered by thoughts that are completely baseless and irrational. By pausing for a moment, you can assess the validity and usefulness of your thoughts – and weigh them against other information – *before* attaching negative labels to them. In essence, you're saying, *I can change my mind!* Remember that feelings are fickle, fleeting, and benign.

Here's another approach. Allow yourself to "let go" of a feeling without judging it at all. Your response to a feeling could be, *I don't have to understand this feeling, and I don't have to take action. Knowing that this feeling is harmless, I am letting it dissolve.*

7. Manage your disappointment

Disappointment triggers a mix of feelings. Many people with depression cannot tolerate even the smallest disappointment. Moreover, a depressed mind tends to exaggerate the magnitude of a disappointment. As the proverb points out, a molehill is made into a mountain. And yes, a depressed mind reinforces thoughts of inadequacy and worthlessness. Fortunately, it's possible to manage your disappointments.

First, identify the disappointment and how you feel about it. Then ask: What would you hope for if you weren't afraid of being disappointed again? Next, reflect on your feelings without trying to change them ... *you didn't get what you wanted in this particular situation. That's disappointing!* Acknowledge the reality that you've lost something you wanted. Validate that feeling – because it's normal to experience sadness after a loss. Finally, decide what to do next. Ask, *What do I need to do in order to move forward with my life?* Hint: Forgiveness is always a wise choice.

8. You have the power to choose

Depression tends to narrow your field of vision. As a result, you focus on your own problems and fail to see other aspects of life. And of course, the world is shrouded in negativity. Still, it's up to you to decide how to perceive what is happening at any given time. You hold the power to view the world through a lens of optimism. And as you consciously change your thoughts from negative to positive, your feelings improve as well.

Instead of being reactional, you become intentional. In short, you become more open-minded and less judgmental. As you practice letting go of judgment, you'll experience longer periods of inner peace. And as an added bonus, you'll have a greater sense of safety and well-being.

9. Not everything is about you

If you're depressed, then you're likely to be self-centered. You're likely to think that every annoying thing that happens was specifically designed to torture you. So here's a reality check: Most events and situations have absolutely nothing to do with you. That means you don't always need to fix a problem that you didn't create. You might even realize that other people have problems too. It can be a relief to learn that you haven't been singled out for punishment, either by God or anyone else.

Are you ready for one more revelation? Try this: You don't have to take life so seriously. In fact, you might even find situations where you can laugh at yourself. Yes, life has serious moments; and of course, there *will* be problems. But perhaps you overestimate the size of your problems or, for that matter, your own importance. Take the time needed to honestly evaluate each obstacle that comes your way. If a barrier turns out to be imaginary, dismiss it. If it's real, find a solution – one that can be broken down into small, manageable steps. If you need help with the problem solving part, consider reaching out to a close friend or trusted coworker.

★★★

Closing reflection ...

Because life is dynamic, your environment – including your work environment – is always changing. Yet, as an intelligent and mindful caregiver, you can adapt and prosper within any landscape. Today's lesson offered a wide range of effective interventions that will help you manage anxiety, stress, and burnout. Review them from time to time. Most importantly, use them when needed.

Take a moment to identify your strengths – your personal attributes – that are empowering you to thrive as a hospice caregiver. Write them down. Study them. Be proud of them. They are true and real – and they are an important part of who you are!

★★★

DAY SEVEN

LOVE

> Love is the highest goal to which we can aspire. In truth, the salvation of humanity is through love and in love. *Viktor Frankl*

★★★

First available in Europe during the1950s, thalidomide became a popular sedative. Soon, doctors learned that the new drug relieved symptoms of morning sickness and, as a result, it was prescribed to pregnant women around the world. No one knew that thalidomide would cause catastrophic problems to developing babies, including heart conditions and limb deformities. In Great Britain alone, about 2,000 babies were affected, with roughly half of them dying within six months. Even the infants who lived to celebrate their first birthday had a shortened life expectancy. And because of their significant disabilities – missing or abnormal arms, hands, legs, and feet – the lives of these children, and of their parents and siblings, were anything but normal.

Just ask the family of Rosie Moriarty, who was born near London in 1962. Each of her stub-like arms had a tiny, two-fingered hand. Her legs ended above the knee, and her two feet featured a total of thirteen miniature toes. While growing up, Rosie faced countless obstacles and dilemmas. Schools, for example, weren't prepared or equipped to educate students confined to wheelchairs. So Rosie and her family were constantly searching for new ways to cope. Somehow, they persevered. After graduating from high school, Rosie presented workshops on equality training to schools and businesses.

She eventually married, and Rosie and her husband became the proud parents of a son, James. Her autobiography *Four Fingers and Thirteen Toes* includes the following statement: "It's almost as if I have no arms or legs at all. But for as long as I can remember, I've campaigned to be treated like everybody else, and I've refused to let thalidomide stop me from living my life."

Despite extraordinary life challenges, Rosie made a deliberate and profound choice: to *not* be a victim. And by rejecting victimhood, her life was blessed with meaning and purpose. She didn't wallow in self-pity, nor did she withdraw from the world and live in misery. Instead, Rosie chose to drink fully from the cup of life – she chose to love herself.

★★★

The BBC television series *Call the Midwife* has gained a large following in both England and America. The actors wear period appropriate wardrobe, and the scripts reflect the culture and values of the time. Season Five includes an episode that chronicles the birth defects attributed to thalidomide. In fact, the show's producers hired Rosie Moriarty as a consultant to ensure that the complex issues were presented accurately and fairly. This wonderfully crafted episode depicts London's East End in 1961 and includes a remarkable scene ...

Laura, the mother of two boys, gives birth to her third child, a baby girl. An attending nurse, spotting the newborn's deformities, whisks the baby away. Viewers learn that the little girl has virtually no arms or hands, and her legs and feet are abnormal as well. Over the next few days, excuses are given as to why Laura cannot meet and hold her new daughter: Baby needs rest; baby must be kept warm; baby is being fed; and so on. Finally, a nurse explains to Laura that her daughter was born with complications, but no details are given. Soon thereafter, the baby is swaddled in a blanket and laid in a bassinet. A nurse escorts Laura into a small, stark room, and points to the bassinet. The nurse leaves and closes the door. Mother and daughter are alone.

Silently approaching her baby, Laura sees a normal head and an adorable face peering upward. A joyful mother carefully lifts her child and holds her for the first time. And their love — the special bond that formed in the womb — is rekindled. Then, ever so gently, Laura unwraps the blanket, not knowing what to expect. Laura's eyes grow wide. Next — a quiet gasp, a furrowed brow, and a look of sadness. Yet, it's an unselfish sadness tied to the pain that her baby might be feeling, and it lasts only a moment. Gently and tenderly, Laura presses the baby to her chest: holding and rocking her, cradling and comforting her. Laura embraces her child so that mom's heart and baby's heart are as close as possible. At that moment, two souls are joined as one; and with eyes closed, Laura sees her precious daughter as she truly is: whole and perfect.

★★★

In the human experience, is there anything greater than the love which a mother offers unconditionally to her newborn child? Is this as close as we can come to Divine love?

Young children have no opinions on what is normal or expected. They just want to be safe and nurtured and loved. How might a child be both imperfect *and* perfect?

Are there sounds more joyous and pure than those of young children on a playground?

★★★

From God's perspective, your earthly job is to expand your faith and elevate your consciousness by growing in trust and gaining wisdom. One of the better ways to achieve this lofty goal is choosing to love — or forgive — all that life offers you, everyone and everything, without exception. You can choose to embrace the holy, the good, and the beautiful even as you endure the profane, the bad, and the ugly. The work is simple, but not easy.

★★★

Since the dawn of human history, men have been killing one another. Murder and war are firmly entrenched in the human condition. If, for example, a migrating tribe encountered unfamiliar people who looked, acted, or thought differently, tribal leaders might conclude, *They can't be trusted. We must kill them.* If a wandering tribe came upon a nation whose people practiced strange rituals or spoke a foreign language, tribal leaders might say, *They could rape our women and slaughter our children. We will go to war with them.* And yes, deadly disputes also arose between individuals and among groups of the same tribe. Violence and mayhem have been around for a long while, and they continue to plague humanity today.

Fortunately, our history has a flip side. While some tribes were at war, others were engaged in trade. While some nations were intent on killing, others were focused on peacefully sharing their language and culture. Though some individuals sought revenge, others chose to forgive. Though some tribes remained bitter enemies, others formed helpful alliances – partnerships that promoted trust and prosperity. Ultimately, it is love which nurtures and sustains us. Love quietly brings people together. Love helps us see the good in those who, at first glance, seem so different. Love heals and unifies and reminds us that we are all made in the image of one Creator.

★★★

Much like life, love is always changing, adapting, and evolving. An infatuation may escalate to a romance. A romantic love might change to a nurturing love. Yesterday's dear friend may become tomorrow's life partner. And a life partner's love might evolve to a caregiver's love.

Still, no matter how it is expressed or how it may change, it is love in all its glory!

★★★

In this world, it often seems like the more you give, the less you have. Yet, there's an uplifting exception; for with love, the more you give the more you receive.

★★★

Love is embracing every situation that comes your way.

Love is seeing God's face in everyone you meet.

Love is finding mercy in chaos.

Love is living your life with unbridled passion.

Love is disallowing hardship to steal your crown.

★★★

Teach only love, for that is what you are. *ACIM*

★★★

Sometimes, love is placing the needs of another ahead of your own needs.

★★★

It is love which joins and holds people together.

★★★

A relationship built on innocence and purity is our greatest human expression.

★★★

Holy relationships are always founded on love; and when anointed by God, loving relationships bring heaven to earth.

★★★

God *is* love. And as a child of God, made in his image, love is the very essence of who you are. Nevertheless, love is a mystery, for it cannot be fully defined. It cannot be entirely explained or understood. You know intuitively that love, though it may be predicted, cannot be controlled or manipulated. You know instinctively that love might be suppressed, but never extinguished. Though it bends, love does not break. And in your heart you know that love is nurtured through forgiveness. Having no true opposite, love unveils the illusion of polarities. Yet, there is a paradox: for love is both the lamb *and* the lion; it is the rose, but also the thorn. Love is both the calm *and* the storm; the sweet *and* the bitter. Love is exquisitely free, yet it flourishes in bonds of devotion. Love never punishes, yet it's the foundation of justice. Love is a witness for truth, yet it doesn't judge. By never condemning, love remains innocent. Love conquers by surrendering, and it rules by lifting up.

Inspired by Glenda Green

★★★

More on love ...

Is there an ultimate declaration of love? Perhaps it is risking one's own life while trying to save the life of another. First responders routinely confront such scenarios, as do troops serving in war zones. That said, it's remarkable how often an unwitting passerby is at the right place and time to help save someone's life.

Kindness elevates human consciousness and, thereby, transforms the world. Indeed, expressions of love are the only way to improve the human condition.

When love is nurtured within a sacred space, there is reason to hope for a better world.

Expressions of love include a calm presence, a gentle touch, and affirming words.

Love is demonstrated by attentive listening, by keeping an open mind, and by giving and receiving gifts.

Love and joy form an unbreakable bond. When you give love, you receive joy. The more love you give, the more joy you receive – and your heart is filled with the peace of God.

Hope, faith, trust, patience, virtue, integrity, and perseverance: all of these are born of love.

As you grow in love, it becomes easier to recognize what is real, what is true, what is good, and what is beautiful. Then, you're better equipped to separate the meaningful from the meaningless.

People share many commonalities: birth and death, thirst and hunger; we laugh, we cry; we bleed, we hurt; we grieve and suffer; we create and celebrate; we love and forgive; we grow and learn; we help, we serve; we make choices – both wise and foolish. Unity celebrates things that are alike, and respects things that are different. Love and unity are joined as one. They cannot be separated any more than light can be separated from the sun.

★★★

A Caregiver's Search for Love

Despite the chaos and tumult you see in our world, love is alive and thriving. Regardless of the fear and pain you witness or experience, love is abundant and flourishing. In truth, evidence of love is all around you.

Love is found by ...

looking deeply into the eyes of a child,

looking fondly at the smile of a partner,

looking closely at the pulse of a patient,

and by looking warmly at the face of a stranger.

Love is ...

nurturing hope as you walk with the wounded,

rekindling joy as you journey with the grieving,

restoring faith as you comfort the sick,

and instilling peace as you serve the dying.

Love is ...

seeing goodness in the unexpected,

finding wholeness in the broken,

noticing beauty in the ordinary,

and discovering grace in the shadows of a tragedy.

★★★

Peace and joy, helpfulness and thoughtfulness, honoring and cherishing, thankfulness and hopefulness, caring and nurturing, kindness and forgiveness – all are expressions of love. And as each loving expression unfolds on earth, heaven rejoices!

★★★

Closing reflection ...

How might you grow in love and faith during a season of pain and hardship?

Reflect on how a parent demonstrates his or her love for a child. What is it that makes someone a more loving parent?

Think about some of the loving couples that you know. What makes their relationships so special? How do they express their love to one another? Are their signs of affection demonstrated in big ways or small ways?

As a couple grows older, it's not uncommon for one of the partners to become a caregiver for the other. This sudden change of roles adds stress to a relationship. What are some of the physical and emotional challenges faced by someone who's providing care for a partner? As for the partner who is receiving care, how might he or she be troubled by this change? What empowers a relationship to withstand the strain of care giving?

When you love someone, is it a sacrifice to place his or her needs above your own? Why or why not?

Think about your typical day at home. Describe the expressions of love that you encounter regularly.

As a hospice caregiver, you provide comfort and support. You are kind and helpful. You offer respect and dignity. You are mindful and attentive. You listen to stories. You manage pain. You offer assurance and affirmation. Indeed, you are an overflowing vessel of love!

Love is the one reality and the single truth. Everything else is a distracting illusion.

★★★

DAY EIGHT

FORGIVENESS

To forgive is to set a prisoner free and discover
that the prisoner was you. *Lewis B. Smedes*

★★★

Hardly a day goes by without a disturbance of some kind, an annoying event that triggers anger. Often, it's something trivial and, therefore, quickly forgotten. But when people are hurt more deeply, healing takes longer. They might ask, *When will my pain go away? How can I cope?* Such thoughts are normal, of course, and offering forgiveness is the best remedy. But occasionally, a betrayal is so stunning and unexpected that life is completely – and perhaps permanently – turned upside-down. And yes, extreme events prompt more complicated questions: *Are some things just too horrible to forgive? Is it possible to love someone who personifies evil?*

Kerri Rader grew up in a suburb of Wichita, Kansas. Her mom, Paula was a housewife and her dad, Dennis worked as a city inspector. Dennis took Kerri and her older brother, Brian on fishing and camping trips. Their family attended a local Lutheran church, and they celebrated Thanksgiving, Christmas, and birthdays just like everyone else on the street. Kerri's childhood was happy. Looking back on those years, she said, "I grew up adoring my dad. He was the sunshine of my life." On Kerri's wedding day, Dennis walked her down the aisle.

By 2005, Kerri and her husband were living in Michigan. She was twenty-six years old and worked as a substitute teacher. On the morning of February 25th, a special agent with the FBI knocked on her door. Kerri learned that her father had been arrested and charged in connection with ten murders. After the agent left, Kerri was stunned. She began to wonder if her whole life had been a lie. Was it true that her dad was a serial killer? Kerri's mind took turns defending, and then doubting, her father's innocence.

Mike Clark, the family's pastor, visited Dennis in jail. The following day, he confessed. Dennis provided details that only the killer could know. Moreover, he talked about his crimes with an arrogance that shocked law enforcement veterans. Dennis was sentenced to live the rest of his natural life in a maximum-security prison. Kerri ended all communication with her father. She despised him.

In 2007, Kerri sought help from Sue Parker, a psychotherapist. Parker learned that Kerri had good people around her, including support from her husband, close friends, and her minister. Having been devastated to a degree which only God could comprehend, Kerri was, from Parker's perspective, remarkably healthy and strong. Still, Kerri had struggled through some terrifying nights. She recalls, "In my dreams, I would fight with my dad, never understanding why he did those terrible things. I was fearful and angry. Sometimes I was fighting for my life, frantically trying to convince people that it wasn't my fault – *that I hadn't committed those crimes*." Parker pointed out that Dennis also had a good side. In truth, there were times when he really was a caring father. Parker hinted that, one day, Kerri might begin to feel sorry for her dad. And if she did, that would be okay.

A few months later, Kerri found the courage to talk to her therapist about another dream. In this one, she felt God's presence. What's more, Kerri received a message that gently guided her in a positive direction:

You have a father problem. You have trust and obedience problems. You trusted and obeyed your earthly father, and he hurt you profoundly. Now, you're withdrawing from me. Let's fix that.

For the first time, Kerri started thinking about forgiving her dad – not to help him, but to ease her own suffering. Kerri realized that she only knew the man who had watched over her and kept her safe. She had never met the man who was a convicted killer; she had never known that man. After five years of silence, she wrote a letter to her father. Kerri told him that, while she would never forget his unspeakable crimes or be at peace with them, she *was* at peace with the dad who raised and cared for her. She gave him updates on her life and shared stories about the grandchildren he would never see. Kerri finished by writing, "I don't think I will ever visit you, but know that I have found a way to love you again."

Adapted from an interview by Roy Wenzl

★★★

Forgiveness doesn't mean condoning and excusing irresponsible or criminal behavior. Forgiveness doesn't mean that you were not hurt, or that you're no longer hurting. Forgiveness doesn't mean offering friendship to an abuser. And forgiveness doesn't mean denying the betrayal and pain you've endured. So then, what *is* forgiveness? Forgiveness is reaffirming one's identity. Forgiveness is re-examining life's meaning. Forgiveness is letting go of past wounds and grievances. Forgiveness is releasing bitter feelings and thoughts of revenge. Forgiveness is moving on to the here and now. Forgiveness is rediscovering moments of happiness. And finally, forgiveness is celebrating your newfound freedom.

★★★

Regardless of Divine forgiveness, evil choices bring severe consequences.

★★★

You needn't feel ashamed of your feelings, nor should you deny them. Still, feelings are transient; they come and go. And most importantly, you can choose to change your mind about things. You can change your perception of the events and circumstances that shape your feelings.

★★★

Forgiveness changes everything. Let's say, for example, that a loved one has betrayed you. Feelings of anger and sadness are sure to follow. But your feelings don't hurt the betrayer, they hurt you – by disrupting your inner peace. When you forgive the betrayer, your sadness and anger begin to subside, and life starts getting better. *You* benefit from this change, not the betrayer. Therefore, the saints and sages are right: Forgiveness is a treasured gift that you receive the very moment you pass it on!

★★★

Forgiveness is an intentional outreach, a spiritual experience shared among God, another, and oneself. Although the language can be simple, the words must be heartfelt. When you've done something you regret, say to that person ...

I'm sorry, please forgive me.

Then, when you're alone, reach out to God and say ...

Gracious God, I ask you for forgiveness.

And when someone offers you an apology, say ...

My friend, I forgive you.

Practice these words, for they are powerful and healing. Embrace them as family, and say them often.

★★★

Self-forgiveness is yet another important part of the journey. Here's a quick look at what self-forgiveness is and isn't.

Self-forgiveness ...

is *not* condoning your behavior and choices.

is *not* blaming someone else for your mistake.

is *not* encouraging you to repeat the mistake.

is *not* denying that you hurt someone.

is *not* denouncing your need to make amends.

Self-forgiveness ...

is offering mercy to oneself.

is a healing process that takes time.

is letting go of the past.

is releasing your pain, guilt, and shame.

is letting go of your self-loathing.

is rejecting victimhood.

★★★

The following, five-step forgiveness model is recommended by therapist, Heather Carlile. Study it carefully, and perhaps her guidelines will help you work through a current or future forgiveness issue. This introspective process is designed for occasions when you've been hurt by someone.

Step One: Uncovering the Injury

- Identify what was said or done, or maybe what *wasn't* said or done.
- How did this injury make you feel?
- What did you say or do in response to this injury?

Step Two: Preparing to Forgive

- You are ready to stop expressing anger.
- You are willing to release thoughts of revenge and punishment.
- You accept the pain and dismiss the suffering.

Step Three: Rebuilding Safety

- You take responsibility for your thoughts and feelings.
- You no longer blame someone else for your beliefs and judgments.
- You do not perceive yourself as a victim.

Step Four: Surrendering and Releasing

- You surrender any feelings of guilt, shame, or hopelessness.
- You let go of fear, resentment, jealousy, and hatred.

Step Five: Looking Ahead

- You open your heart to empathy and compassion.
- You discover a spiritual lesson in your forgiveness journey.
- You relinquish your desire to be faultless.
- You dismiss the desire to control your relationships.

Closing reflection ...

Think about your interactions at work. Identify a time when your feelings were hurt by either a coworker or a patient. Have you offered forgiveness to that person? If not, can you forgive him or her now?

Next, try to remember an occasion where a close friend or family member has hurt your feelings. Is it harder or easier to forgive someone you love? Why?

Have you forgiven that close friend or family member? If not, can you forgive him or her now?

Everything you get angry about has occurred in the past. Maybe it was something that happened decades ago; or perhaps it occurred just a moment ago. Either way, you can't change it. Just bless it, and let it go.

Though it will never change the past, forgiveness *can* change the future.

★★★

DAY NINE

VIKTOR FRANKL

To live is to suffer; to survive is to find meaning
in suffering. *Friedrich Nietzsche*

★★★

From 1942 through 1945, Austrian psychiatrist Viktor Frankl was held captive in a morbid series of Nazi concentration camps. His typical day started just before dawn, when prisoners were assembled for a roll-call by number. Then, Frankl reported to his assigned work group, marched from camp to the project site, spent the entire day doing hard manual labor, and marched back to camp at sunset. It was an exhausting routine that demoralized many of the prisoners. Cruel guards, rancid food, and filthy, cramped living conditions added to the misery. Separated from their loved ones and with virtually no chance of escape, most of the men lost hope – and their will to live. Frankl could see it in their vacant eyes: the death stare. Countless men succumbed to the ravages of disease and starvation. But did a broken spirit hasten their demise?

Frankl witnessed *and* endured unimaginable suffering during his incarceration. Immersed in squalor, he watched as vibrant men were slowly reduced to emaciated skeletons. And he, too, walked that path. Yet, he also observed incredible acts of kindness – unexpected charity offered by prisoners and guards alike. He learned that one German officer used his own money to buy medicine for the camp's infirmary. And Frankl was awestruck by prisoners who disregarded their own needs while addressing the needs of fellow prisoners. These special men not only comforted the sick, they shared their meager food rations with those who were too weak to work. After living in four different camps, Frankl noticed a pattern: Some men behaved like savage animals, while others kept their human dignity and respect. Moreover, he knew that every man had made a conscious choice on how to respond to the camp environment. He wondered, *What drives a man to choose good over evil?*

In an uncanny sequence of events, Frankl lived long enough to be liberated by American soldiers. Shortly thereafter, he learned that his parents, brother, and pregnant wife had perished. Frankl, while processing his personal tragedies, concluded that people cannot avoid suffering, but they can choose how to cope with it. People can find meaning in their suffering, and move forward with renewed purpose. Frankl shares his compelling journey in *Man's Search for Meaning* – one of the most influential books of the twentieth century. His insights and theories on human nature continue to influence today's therapists.

★★★

More important than our search for pleasure (as promoted by Freud), and more essential than our quest for power (as advanced by Nietzsche),

Viktor Frankl argued that humans are driven by a motivation to find meaning in life. With this in mind, Frankl developed logotherapy, an entirely new school of psychotherapy. Here's an overview of its principles:

- Regardless of the circumstances, life has meaning – even as we're facing hardship and misery.
- What drives our will to live? According to Frankl, it's to discover a meaning in one's life.
- We have an opportunity to find meaning in our activities, in our experiences, and in the attitude we adopt while facing unavoidable suffering.

Frankl explains that everything can be taken from us, except how we choose to perceive a given set of circumstances. Although he warns against pursuing hedonism and materialism, Frankl states that, when possible, suffering should be avoided. Moreover, he believes that a person does not necessarily have to suffer in order to find meaning in life.

★★★

Prior to the insights of Abraham Maslow, psychologists defined people solely by their abnormalities. So in this sense, Maslow's work was truly groundbreaking, for it focused on the positive aspects of human behavior, needs, and desires. Yet, his paradigm lacked a spiritual dimension; and that's why some of Maslow's contemporaries, including Viktor Frankl, founded the school of Transpersonal Psychology. In some ways, this progression mirrors the contributions of Carl Jung, who added Divinity to the seminal work of Sigmund Freud.

Transpersonal Psychology teaches that one's identity extends beyond the individual and personal to encompass all life and phenomena within the universe. It is a broader sense of self that includes spiritual and mystical experiences, and even altered states of consciousness. It suggests that there's an interconnectedness among life, consciousness, and the cosmos; and that each life form is, in truth, part of a greater whole.

Both Maslow and Frankl acknowledged the transformative qualities of a "peak" experience, defined as a profoundly exhilarating and elevating event that produces holistic ecstasy. However, Maslow believed that a peak experience propels an individual to reach his or her full potential; while for Frankl, such an experience leads an individual to discover life's meaning.

★★★

Viktor Frankl: Thoughts and reflections ...

Suffering completely fills the conscious mind, without regard to whether the pain is great or small. So it follows that a trifling thing holds the potential to trigger immense joy.

Outside forces can take away all that you possess, except for one thing: the freedom to choose how you respond to what happens in life. This freedom makes life meaningful and purposeful.

The death camp prisoners who let go of their moral and spiritual selves eventually fell victim to the camp's degenerating influences. A few men accepted their circumstances as an opportunity to achieve an inner triumph. But most of the prisoners ignored this challenge and simply chose to vegetate.

There are but two races of men in the world: the decent and the indecent. Both are found everywhere; they penetrate all groups of society. No single group consists entirely of decent or indecent people.

The rift dividing good from evil, which goes through all men, extends deep into the human soul.

Live as if you were living for the second time, and as if you had acted wrongly the first time.

Love is the only way to fully grasp another human being. You cannot know the very essence of another person unless you love him.

People have no right to do wrong, even if wrong has been done to them.

Try to make responsible choices, ones that are right, moral, and decent. Then, accept ownership of your choices and their consequences.

That which gives light must endure burning.

Our capacity to love is humanity's salvation.

Between stimulus and response there is a space. In that space you have the power to choose your response. And in your response lies your growth and freedom.

A search for meaning is life's primary motivation. You can find meaning by doing a kind deed, by loving someone, by forgiving someone, or by creating something – such as a work of art. You can also find meaning as you experience goodness, truth, and beauty. Life's meaning is always changing, and you don't have to suffer to discover it.

A human being is not one thing among others; *things* determine each other, but *human beings* are self-determining.

Life and freedom bring responsibility.

A positive attitude empowers you to endure suffering and disappointment, and it also enhances enjoyment and satisfaction. A negative attitude intensifies pain and undermines pleasure. Negativity may well lead to depression or even physical illness. Within the limits of endowment and environment, you become what you make of yourself.

★★★

"A few days after my liberation, I took a long walk in the country. As I passed through a flowering meadow, larks rose to the sky and I listened to their joyous songs. There was no one for miles around; there was nothing but the wide earth and sky, the larks, and the freedom of space. I stopped, looked up, and fell to my knees. There was but one thought in my mind: I had called out to God from my narrow prison, and at this moment, he had answered me. On that day, in that hour, my new life started. Step by step I progressed, until I became a human being again." *Viktor Frankl*

★★★

Closing reflection ...

Look back on your recent activities and experiences. Which ones have added meaning to *your* life? Why?

Identify the people who add meaning and purpose to your life. Why do you have such strong feelings for them?

And for those who have died ...

Do you believe that, in the afterlife, the people you cherish are forever safe and loved?

Is it possible to both mourn *and* celebrate someone's death?

Do you accept that your life will never be quite the same without these special people?

Is it possible to honor the dead by rediscovering joy in the here and now?

★★★

DAY TEN

MUSIC

The earth has music for those who listen. *William Shakespeare*

★★★

Scholars say that music is an art form of sound and silence unfolding within the structure of time. Its common elements include pitch (melody and harmony), rhythm (tempo and meter), dynamics (loudness and softness), and timbre (texture and color). And because it's the product of vibrations, sound waves, and frequencies, music is governed by the same laws of physics that rule our universe. Fast vibrations produce high frequencies that, in turn, create thin, high-pitched sounds. Meanwhile, slower vibrations make the low frequencies that produce low-pitched, deep sounds. That's why a cello, with longer and thicker strings, makes lower pitched sounds than its smaller counterpart, the violin. Following the same principle, women usually have smaller vocal chords than men and, as a result, their voices are higher pitched.

Still, a scientific analysis of music doesn't begin to capture its essence. Music is deeply entrenched in human minds and hearts. It mirrors our culture and expresses our feelings. In truth, music touches the soul. Contemporary spiritual teachers suggest that love is a manifestation of high frequency vibrations. And if this is so, then music and love are intrinsically, and forever, entwined. Frequently integrated with other art forms, music adds harmony to poetry and rhythm to movement. Music plays a key role in both religious and secular ceremonies and celebrations: birthdays, weddings, funerals, graduations, and so on. Music – whether it's a humble lullaby, or a grandiose Mass – can lighten burdens, brighten moods, lessen pain, and trigger joy.

There are many genres and styles of music, from jazz to rock and roll; from gospel to bluegrass; from classical to hip-hop, and everything in between. It isn't that certain kinds of music are *better* than others, they're just *different* from one another. Depending on what you're searching for, music can leave you feeling carefree or reflective, relaxed or energized, introverted and subdued, or bold and adventurous. By God's grace, music is immensely diverse. No matter where you go in the world, people are creating and performing music that's uniquely tied to their local culture. Caribbean and Eastern music, for instance, not only have entirely different melodic, harmonic, and rhythmic qualities, they feature contrasting instrumentation as well.

Let's not forget the noteworthy "behind the scene" stories tied to music. For example, men and women spend decades mastering the instrumental and vocal skills required to perform grand orchestral and choral music. Moreover, many of the stringed instruments used by today's professional musicians were hand-crafted hundreds of years ago. And only recently have we developed the technology to record a marvelous concert and listen to it again and again with sound, clarity, depth, and balance that rival the live performance.

And yes, music is also therapeutic. Research has proven that spoken language is processed by one part of the human brain, while music is processed by a different part. Therefore, people with brain disorders, such as Alzheimer's disease, often respond better to music, than they do to spoken words. Music therapy utilizes creative interventions – live performances, sing-alongs, recordings, and hands-on activities – that are customized to achieve optimal outcomes. Music therapy ...

Reduces fear and anxiety.

Elevates the responsiveness of older adults, especially those with dementia.

Calms people who are struggling with shortness of breath.

Helps manage pain.

Improves communication for people functioning in the autism spectrum.

Promotes weight gain and healthier sleep patterns among infants born prematurely.

Enhances motor function for adults with Parkinson's disease.

★★★

Musical notation is a unique and ingenious marriage of language, mathematics, and design that unites divided nations and cultures.

A wide variety of musical tones – generated by brass, woodwind, percussion, keyboard, and stringed instruments – blend harmoniously, as though they were all born of the same loving mother.

Like a familiar, intoxicating fragrance, music can spark memories of treasured people and precious moments.

Music is an inspired blend of physics, mathematics, and love.

★★★

Nature is constantly creating its own music, pulse, and vibe – a wonderful mix of improvised elegance and synchronized chaos.

In a meadow, listen intently for buzzing bees and singing birds.

In a canyon, you might hear rushing water or whistling wind.

On a farm, be prepared for crowing roosters, grunting pigs, and mooing cows.

Near a pond, you're likely to hear splashing fish or croaking frogs.

In a jungle, listen for quarreling monkeys, roaring tigers, and trumpeting elephants.

At the shore, you might hear crashing waves or screeching gulls.

In the woods, be alert for babbling brooks, creaking trees, growling bears, and rustling leaves.

On a plain, dark skies are often accompanied by rolling thunder and pounding rain.

At night, a wilderness campsite could be serenaded by hooting owls, chirping crickets, or howling wolves.

If you were listening to sounds beneath the sea, you might hear chatty dolphins and moaning whales.

Look to the sky in order to spot ranting starlings, honking geese, and quacking ducks.

And at your feet, you just might discover a purring kitten or a whimpering puppy.

★★★

Bucket lists appear to be growing in popularity. So with that in mind, here are eight musical selections that you simply *must* listen to, preferably decades before "kicking the bucket." In terms of artistic creativity, these masterworks are among humanity's finest achievements; and the recommended performances are absolutely stellar. The play length is provided so that you can set aside enough time to enjoy each of these ageless treasures at your leisure and without interruption.

Mass in B Minor, composed by Johann Sebastian Bach (1685 – 1750); conducted by Philippe Herreweghe; featuring the Collegium Vocale Gent; recorded in 2011; playing time 102 minutes. Bach's rich textures and astonishing counterpoint are captured in acoustical perfection. Angelic vocals soar under Herreweghe's watchful eye, bringing heaven to earth. Technically, it's one of the finest recordings ever produced. Did Bach ever imagine that his music could be performed so elegantly?

The Goldberg Variations, composed by Johann Sebastian Bach (1685 – 1750); recorded in 1955 and remastered by Sony Music in 2002; performed by Canadian piano savant, Glenn Gould; playing time 39 minutes. Most piano virtuosos place their hands above the top of the keyboard, thereby positioning their fingers to *push* the keys down. But Gould, who sits closer to the floor, places his hands near the front edge of the keyboard, thereby allowing his fingers to *pull* the keys down. The result is stunning. Like an exquisite string of pearls, individual notes are identical in shape, tone, and clarity – yet they're perfectly joined to the ones played just before and after. Very few pianists have reached this level of precision and artistry.

Messiah, composed by George Frideric Handel (1685 – 1759); conducted by Robert Shaw; featuring the Atlanta Symphony Orchestra and Chamber Chorus; recorded in 1984; playing time 140 minutes. In this version of the life of Jesus, Maestro Shaw coaxes brilliant performances from both orchestra and chorus. Soloists Sylvia McNair (soprano) and Cornelius Hauptmann (bass) are especially impressive.

Great Mass in C Minor, an unfinished work composed by Wolfgang Amadeus Mozart (1756 – 1791); conducted by John Eliot Gardiner; featuring the Monteverdi Choir; recorded in 1986; playing time 54 minutes. Mozart reaches dazzling new heights, and soprano Sylvia McNair cements her status as a modern-day muse. This Mass is a rich manifestation of truth, beauty, and holiness.

Requiem, composed by Wolfgang Amadeus Mozart (1756 – 1791); conducted by Georg Solti; recorded live at Saint Stephen's Cathedral in 1991; playing time 58 minutes. The skilled baton of Sir Georg guides a flawless performance graced by church bells and Latin liturgy. Mozart died before completing *Requiem*. Yet, this version includes a masterfully composed, posthumous ending that was inspired by Mozart's own handwritten notations.

Mass in C, composed by Ludwig van Beethoven (1770 – 1827); conducted by John Eliot Gardiner; featuring the Monteverdi Choir;

recorded in 1993; playing time 48 minutes. Beethoven demonstrates why the Mass is a sublime musical form – six movements that nourish the soul: Kyrie (Lord have mercy), Gloria (Glory to God in the highest), Credo (I believe in one God), Sanctus (Holy, holy, holy, Lord God of hosts), Benedictus (Blessed is he who comes in the name of the Lord), and Agnus Dei (Lamb of God).

Symphony No. 9, composed by Ludwig van Beethoven (1770 – 1827); conducted by Paavo Jarvi; featuring the Dutch Philharmonic Orchestra; recorded in 2009; playing time 64 minutes. Maestro Jarvi highlights the timpani and pushes the tempo in this exhilarating performance. The composer's innovative format of three instrumental movements followed by a choral finale had never been tried. What's more, Beethoven had lost his hearing before writing this symphony, a classic that will have you jumping for joy!

Stabat Mater, composed by Antonin Dvorak (1841 – 1904); conducted by Robert Shaw; featuring the Atlanta Symphony Orchestra and Chorus; recorded in 1999; playing time 86 minutes. Dvorak was grieving as he composed this piece – three of his children had recently died. Still, he found a way to write music so passionate that it literally brings tears to the eyes of performers and listeners alike. Are there other compositions that match its beauty? Perhaps, but none surpass it.

These are powerful, transformative creations. If you wish, you can leave this divisive world for a short while – as each of the above musical experiences will guide you to a peaceful, healing realm of harmony and oneness. Just choose to listen, and allow it to happen. As Glenn Gould observed, "The purpose of art is not the release of a momentary rush of adrenaline, but rather the gradual, lifelong construction of a state of wonder and serenity."

★★★

It should be noted that Gould recorded Bach's Goldberg Variations again in 1981, twenty-six years after his initial recording. This version was also remastered in 2002, and some view it as a more mature interpretation. Or if you prefer a very recent Bach performance, listen to the one by Great Britain's master pianist, Oliver Poole. His brilliant interpretation of the Goldberg Variations was video-recorded live at the Opus Theater, and is available on YouTube (playing time 45 minutes). A live performance presents daunting challenges to soloists and recording engineers. The most obvious one is that, unlike a studio session, there are no do-overs.

Bonus: Check out Poole's breathtaking performance of Wagner's Ring Cycle Transcription. It's Part Two of the Opus Theater concert, and that video is on YouTube as well (playing time 25 minutes).

A number of the musical compositions listed above are available on YouTube – but perhaps not the recommended performances. Sometimes ebay is an attractive option for purchasing hard-to-find CDs. Just remember that high fidelity sound reproduction will dramatically boost your listening pleasure.

★★★

Closing reflection ...

What kinds of music do you enjoy listening to? How does music affect your mood? Your feelings? Why does music touch your heart? What is it that moves you?

Would an afterlife not include heavenly music? Would there not be angelic choirs creating celestial sounds never before heard by human ears?

★★★

DAY ELEVEN

DEATH AND AFTERLIFE

The pain of parting is nothing to the joy of
meeting again. *Charles Dickens*

★★★

When a loved one dies, you grieve. Intuitively, you know that your
life will never be quite the same. And though it's normal to mourn, it's
also normal for the pain to slowly fade a bit. Ultimately, grief requires
healing; and healing is nurtured through forgiveness. This doesn't mean
you should forget deceased loved ones, or stop missing them, or erase
their memories. It simply means letting go of the past and accepting
the present circumstances. You might need to forgive hurtful things
that were said or done. Or you might need to forgive a loved one just
because he or she has left you behind.

Those who are grief stricken not only endure emotional pain, they
experience physical changes as well. Sometimes called "broken-heart"
syndrome, stress hormones can cause the heart to enlarge which, in
turn, may produce chest pains or shortness of breath. Yet, the possible
threats associated with grief can be even more serious. Studies show
that strokes and heart attacks are more likely to occur in the thirty days
following the death of a loved one. Such a loss is literally a shock to
our health and well-being. Keep in mind that when a loved one dies,
grieving can be postponed, but not erased.

Grief is not depression, but those who are mourning may become
depressed. In fact, depression is frequently found in cases of "complicated
grief"– a term describing people burdened by debilitating hopelessness,
despondency, and sadness that lasts for six months or longer. Complicated
grief has been linked to hypertension, drug and alcohol abuse, and
suicidal thoughts and behavior. Those who are struggling with profound
and lasting grief have not yet forgiven the past, nor have they genuinely

accepted their loss of a loved one. They resist living in the present moment and, as a result, they're unable to move on with their lives – they're unable to regain normal psychological and social functioning.

For caregivers, the death of a patient is typically less traumatic than the death of a family member or a close friend. Still, you often grow close to your patients, and your attachment – your love for them – is very real. So yes, there will be sadness when a patient dies. Moreover, the sheer number and frequency of these deaths will amplify your sense of loss. Of course, witnessing a difficult death – for instance, when a patient bleeds out – is particularly disturbing. Talk to your supervisor or a counselor after an event like this. Talking about the experience will help you process it, and sharing your feelings with someone you trust will foster healing.

★★★

Though there are always exceptions, life generally unfolds in a predictable series of chapters. There's an arrival chapter followed by a childhood chapter. Then, an adolescent chapter segues to an adult chapter. Perhaps a marriage chapter is next, and that may lead to a child-raising chapter. Usually, there's a career chapter, a chapter of good health, a chapter of decline, an empty nest chapter, a retirement chapter, and finally: a chapter that features your departure. Frequently, the chapters overlap or progress simultaneously. Certain chapters – marriage, for instance – might be repeated several times. Most chapters include both trials and triumphs. The end of a chapter may, on occasion, be sad. But other times, you can't wait to turn the page and begin a new season. After enduring a painful chapter, you can always hope the next one will be a bit easier. Nevertheless, as you look back on your life and your legacy, you might find that there were hidden blessings in every chapter, even the most difficult ones.

★★★

You have but one life. Yet, that one life has many chapters.

★★★

Each man, woman, and child is blessed by awareness. A researcher might refer to this awareness as consciousness. A physician may call it a life force. A shaman might identify it as spirit, and a priest will call it a soul. Regardless of the label, this part of you is eternal and is, therefore, untouched by your body's demise. This sacred part of you doesn't grow old or weak, tired or sick. Your spirit – your soul – is the essence of your true identity, the part that cannot be harmed.

★★★

While in her London home, Annie vividly remembers clutching her chest, coughing, and struggling for breath: "I had never felt anything like that before. It was as though my trachea was blocked. I couldn't inhale. It was a terrifying sensation." At the same time, Annie experienced a compelling urge to call the hospital in America where her mother had been admitted. Annie, still gasping for breath, dialed the number and asked to be connected to her mother's room. She recalls, "My sister answered and was surprised to hear my voice. She was just about to call and let me know that mom was dying. My sister put the phone to my mother's ear, and I was able to tell her that I loved her. I told her it was okay to let go. While my sister was still holding the phone, mom took her last breath."

Annie explained, "Later, I found out that mom had been coughing and fighting to breathe for about thirty minutes before I called the hospital." Was Annie's shortness of breath just a coincidence? She doesn't think so: "There's no doubt that mom was reaching out to me across thousands of miles. She wanted the chance to say goodbye, and that was her way to make it happen." Having investigated similar scenarios, researchers call this phenomenon an "empathetic death experience."

★★★

Hazel had promised to stop by on Saturday and visit her friend, Sally. At the appointed time, Hazel climbed the porch steps, walked to Sally's front door and rang the bell. Unexpectedly, a man opened the door. He smiled and said, "Hi, I'm Arnold." It turned out that he and Sally were cousins, and Hazel felt an immediate attraction. Looking back, she remembered thinking, *I like this man!*

Sure enough, they dated, fell madly in love, and were married. Their devoted partnership lasted fifty-seven years. When Arnold was diagnosed with cancer, Hazel became his primary caregiver. He quickly realized that his days on earth were numbered. One evening, Arnold motioned Hazel to his bedside. He whispered, "I've always protected you, and I promise to keep you safe. I will always love you." Arnold died later that night.

Every once in a while, an unruly group of teenagers would vandalize Hazel's front yard. These occasional incidents were more annoying than dangerous. But two years after her husband's death, a more serious threat unfolded. Hazel was rudely awakened in the middle of the night. A menacing stranger stood outside her home, banging on the doors and windows. Then, the trespasser tried to open her bedroom widow. Paralyzed by fear, Hazel stayed in bed and closed her eyes. She agonized over what might happen next. But to Hazel's surprise, her fear gave way to an overwhelming stillness and peace. Hazel felt the presence of the person she loved more than anyone: Arnold. While her eyes remained closed, she felt his hand gently stroke her arm. Hazel said, "I don't know who's outside my window." And the voice she new so well replied, "Maybe I'll know who it is." She listened to Arnold's footsteps as he left the bedroom and walked down the hallway. Moments later, the outside banging stopped.

It took Hazel a long time to process and accept what actually happened that night. In the end, she was grateful that Arnold had kept his promise to protect her. And she earnestly prayed that God would forgive her husband for "sneaking out of heaven." Although Hazel lived in that same home for six more years, there were no more threats of intrusion or acts of vandalism.

★★★

Scientists have long known that subatomic particles share an incredible attraction. Moreover, quantum physics includes a mysterious phenomenon called *entanglement*. Here's what happens. If, for example, a laser beam is used to split a photon in half, the two halves somehow stay "connected" even when they are physically separated by a vast distance. As a result, if one-half of a split photon begins to spin – usually because it's being observed – then the "separated" half starts spinning as well. Albert Einstein dubbed this puzzling behavior "eerie." Yet could it be that, after a death, two devoted souls can remain linked? Are kindred spirits, on some level, still joined with their absent companion? Can human bonds somehow span the distance between heaven and earth? And is there a more powerful attractor than love?

★★★

As human beings, we are the only mammals on the planet who are aware that, one day, we shall die.

★★★

As we draw closer to death, God frequently offers gifts of grace. God may, for instance, allow someone to see a glimpse of heaven's beauty – a gentle reminder that there's nothing to fear. Sometimes, God may allow the vision of a deceased family member to appear – a familiar presence that brings comfort and reassurance; a sign that everything is unfolding perfectly.. Other times, a brilliant white light may shine forth, a luminance that promotes healing and a sense of well-being. Or perhaps God may send an angel; for an angel's touch is so tender and comforting. Angels are both loving attendants and vigilant protectors. So it makes sense that heavenly angels are guiding souls across the bridge from here to the hereafter. Would a God of grace not make provisions for a calm, safe journey? And would a God of love not make plans for a joyous homecoming celebration?

★★★

Bedside visions are real. This explains why a patient's eyes may be fixed on a certain spot in the room, and why the patient is reaching out, as if he or she is pointing to someone or something. These visions are not opiate-induced hallucinations, nor are they produced by low blood oxygen levels or brain deterioration.

★★★

The human body gets cancer, but the spirit does not. The body dies, but the spirit does not.

★★★

Once, there was a time before you were; but there shall never be a time when you are not.

★★★

The afterlife is timeless — there are no clocks or calendars. And will there not be limitless opportunities to draw nearer to God?

★★★

When immersed in Divine light and love, it's impossible to feel that someone or something is missing.

★★★

In the bookshelves of the universe, your every thought is recorded. All your words and deeds are meticulously accounted for. Perhaps you're worried these archives will be used to condemn you. Yet in truth, this very evidence shall prove your innocence.

★★★

In the afterlife, you will experience a heightened sense of reality. And as you become oriented to this timeless realm, all earthly pain is quickly forgotten.

★★★

God has created countless physical and metaphysical worlds. And will there not be opportunities to explore them, if you wish? There is, of course, a common thread linking the concrete to the ethereal: All environments offer the chance to grow in love and faith.

★★★

You never stop learning. Yet, in the afterlife, you don't become weary or forlorn. To the contrary, as your journey unfolds, you gain more energy and zeal. Your feet feel lighter and your pace quickens. And just as it is on earth, you continue to blaze a one-of-a-kind trail.

★★★

On this planet, everyone who takes a first breath will inevitably take a last one.

★★★

Is a natural death not as holy as a natural birth? Is a loved one's last breath not as sacred as the first?

★★★

During your transition to the afterlife, you will never lose your awareness or sense of self. In fact, you will feel more alive than ever before – as if you were awakening from a dream.

★★★

Those who survive a near-death experience typically lose their fear of dying. Why might this happen?

★★★

When you're seated in a theater, the curtain rises and a stage appears. When you're approaching death, the veil is lifted and a new world appears.

★★★

Death is but a gentle awakening, a passage which takes you from the shadows to the light.

★★★

The afterlife includes countless opportunities for your love to grow and evolve. As you move from room to room, you remain unaware of higher realms. Yet, as your faith matures, you learn to accept what *is*. You learn to embrace the circumstances which confront you, and be at peace with them. Then, frustration and disappointment can no longer haunt you.

★★★

Shortly before taking your last breath, there's a clear understanding that life continues. At that moment, worry and anxiety are replaced by relief and freedom. Next, you realize that everything is exactly as it should be; and your relief and freedom yield to profound peace and joy. Such is the grace of God!

★★★

In some cultures, a loved one's death is followed by horror, anguish, and gnashing of teeth. In other cultures, that same death will spark a festive celebration complete with music, dancing, and a feast.

★★★

On the physical plane, death is final, absolute, and often tinged with sadness. It is nature's counterpart to birth. Yet, mortality applies only to the body. For on the spirit plane, death is a transition – the end of one experience and the start of a new one. And while endings are bittersweet, beginnings are filled with glorious expectations.

★★★

People usually entertain thoughts of death for just a short time. Otherwise, they may feel overwhelmed. Yet, people who summon the courage to face death's certainty — those who find the strength to examine and to accept their mortality — sometimes receive an unexpected gift: a renewed joy for living. Often, they choose to drink more fully from the cup of life.

★★★

Human beings are creative by nature. In this world, our creative instincts are fulfilled by endeavors such as music, art, theater, design, sculpting, writing, and so on. We pursue these activities with immense passion, and we derive great pleasure from them. Yet, would heaven's opportunities not be exponentially more rewarding? In the afterlife, perhaps love and free will are manifested through creations of unimaginable elegance and complexity.

★★★

What is it to cease breathing but to free the breath from its restless tides; to free one's breath so that it may rise and expand and seek God unencumbered?

Only when you drink from the river of silence shall you begin to sing.

Only when you reach the top of the mountain shall you begin to climb.

And when the earth shall claim your limbs, only then shall you begin to dance.

Kahlil Gibran

★★★

Death is my dear friend, the one who will lead me home to God.

Cardinal Joseph Bernardin

★★★

Isaiah 55:12 promises: You will go out in joy and be led forth in peace; the mountains and hills will burst into song before you, and all the trees of the field will clap their hands.

★★★

Closing reflection ...

God has already prepared a place for you in heaven. Even now, a room awaits you – a safe, restful space for you to heal and to remember your wholeness and perfection.

Imagine a realm of indescribable beauty, a peaceful sanctuary where you bathe in the light of your Creator. Envision a paradise absent of stereotypes. Could it be that, in heaven, there are no earthly names or roles? Perhaps it will no longer be Bob, the husband, dad, and plumber; or Susan, the wife, mom, and lawyer. Instead, picture an environment where you are known simply as a child of God. And in this realm, you enjoy an intimate, eternal connection with all whom you've known and loved.

That which saddens the caterpillar brings joy to the butterfly. Would you be satisfied with a heavenly body made of flesh and bone?

What is your vision of heaven? Of an afterlife? Describe your perfect, eternal setting. What might you experience?

Reflect on your personal views of death and dying. What role do they play in your hospice work? How do they help you cope with the pain that comes from losing a patient? Do your spiritual beliefs help you withstand the relentless drumbeat of death? Why or why not?

★★★

DAY TWELVE

GOD, MEDITATION, AND PRAYER

Prayer is a natural expression of faith, just as
breathing is of life. *Jonathan Edwards*

★★★

Prayer is an opportunity to commune with God, to develop a personal relationship with him. If you wish, you can start a conversation and share your thoughts and feelings. You can ask God for help – for strength, wisdom, guidance, or courage. You can ask for comfort, calmness, and peace. And you needn't say the words out loud, for God always hears the prayers which come from your heart. As you reach out to your Creator more often, you feel closer and more connected to him.

Meditation and reflection are opportunities to open your mind and heart to God. It's the gentle prodding needed to lift the veil of human illusion and discover Divine reality. Contemplative moments help you focus on the meaningful while sorting through an endless parade of distractions. Meditation and reflection guide you to look inward and uncover your true essence. Quiet, solitary time builds patience and trust; it leads to an acceptance of God's will and, thereby, gives the gift of peace.

★★★

Because God is ineffable – beyond what words can describe and minds can comprehend – we find clever ways to mitigate our uncertainty. We use noble, benevolent titles when addressing our Maker: Holy Father, Gracious Lord, Heavenly Comforter, and so on. We assign a gender to God, and we favor human metaphors such as: "I'm in the hands of God" or, "I'll see the face of God." We even saddle God with familiar faults, like jealousy and intolerance. Still, there's nothing wrong with resourceful attempts to make our Creator more approachable. For in truth, nothing pleases God more than your choice to build a close, personal relationship with him.

★★★

As you grow in love and faith, you gain greater clarity of physical and metaphysical realities. You gain a more illuminated vision of God and self. Gradually, it becomes easier to identify truth and to live as God wishes you to live.

★★★

Duke University cardiologist, Mitchell Krucoff chose 150 heart patients to participate in a blind study. Krucoff wanted to see if prayers might promote healing. His findings: After having a heart procedure, the patients who received prayer – in addition to the therapeutic interventions received by everyone – healed twice as fast.

Another Duke University physician, Harold Koenig discovered that his hospitalized patients who received prayer were, on average, able to return home three times sooner than his patients who didn't. Studies have also shown that people who pray daily are forty percent less likely to suffer from a stroke or a heart attack. Indeed, research confirms the efficacy of prayer.

★★★

Prayer and meditation boost your emotional well-being, and studies indicate that emotional stability strengthens the body's immune system. Simply said, spiritual practices actually promote wellness and lessen your risk of illness. So as you pray and meditate, you really *are* fending off those flu viruses!

★★★

Prayer and meditation spark physiological changes. Your heart rate slows down and your blood pressure stabilizes. Muscles relax and tensions ease. Moreover, your brain releases endorphins that promote a sense of safety and well-being.

★★★

God, grant me the serenity to accept the things I cannot change, the courage to change the things I can, and the wisdom to know the difference.

The following exercise is appropriate for situations at work, at home, or in the community:

1. As you witness pain and suffering, ask: Can I change what might unfold?
2. If your answer is *No*, then accept what *is*.
3. If your answer is *Yes*, then ask God for guidance on how you can provide help or comfort in a way that serves the greater good.

★★★

Available in twenty-seven languages, *A Course in Miracles* is nearing its forty-fifth consecutive year in print. As spiritual books go, the *Course* – as it's often called – isn't easy. It can take years of study to grasp some of the more nuanced and layered lessons.

While the lengthy text offers plenty of enigmas, none are more puzzling than the four word declaration: *You need do nothing.* So, what does this concise message actually mean? At first, it appears to chastise the meme which exalts human busyness. And yes, life is very hectic at times. You go here and there. You do this and that. Eventually, you feel guilty whenever a moment of free time arises.

On the gentler side of life, it's more difficult to be thoughtful, kind, and helpful when you're overloaded with things to do and places to go. And it's harder to be caring and compassionate when you're tired and stressed. But in order to gain greater insight on this particular *Course* lesson, let's dig deeper.

When you examine the lives of mystics, prophets, saints, and sages, a distinct pattern emerges. There were periods of time when these special people walked among the masses. There were stretches of time when they were leading, serving, and teaching their brothers and sisters. But there were also occasions when they journeyed to a mountaintop. In other words, these anointed ones were often alone. And it was during such times that their pathway turned inward. Through reflection, prayer, and meditation, they communed with God; and their Divine connections were profoundly healing because they were formed in stillness and solitude.

Globally, sacred texts share a common theme: When searching for God, look deep within your heart. The message is clear. You find peace in sacred solitude; you find renewal in holy silence. At last, the *Course* lesson begins to make sense. The trip that *you* make to the mountaintop can be literal, or figurative. Yet, upon arrival ... you need do nothing.

★★★

Have you ever wondered why God answers some prayers, but not others? Let's be clear. Just because a prayer goes unanswered doesn't mean that God has limits or boundaries. Nor does it mean that there aren't any miracles. Rather, it has more to do with Divine nature. So the next time you ask God for something, remember that, first, it must come from your heart. That is, your prayer must be fueled by love – not hatred, anger, greed, or jealousy. Because God *is* love, he responds to love. And second, your prayer must be rooted in reality, not illusion. In short, because God *is* reality, he only responds to what is real.

For instance, if you and your family are at the beach and your daughter wants you to help her build a sandcastle, you might pause for a moment and silently ask God for inspiration to create a wonderful sandcastle. It's an honest outreach which comes from your heart. Moreover, since it's tied to a real interaction with your child, you have every reason to believe that your prayer will be answered. But what if, at a later date, you visit the beach and ask for God's help in building a sandcastle that you and your family can live in? Is this prayer likely to manifest?

While these beach scenarios may seem trite, bear in mind that, from God's perspective, much of what we pray for is every bit as misguided as the prospect of living in a sandcastle. Perhaps this explains why so many people have wrongly concluded that God doesn't answer prayers – or even worse, that God doesn't exist. There's one more wild card in this equation: Because God may answer your prayer in a way, or at a time, that's completely unexpected, his response could easily go unnoticed. Or then again, his answer could be, "No."

★★★

Would God not recognize the metaphysical as more meaningful than the physical, the supernatural as more real than the natural?

★★★

Although God may not attach value to the same things that are important to you, his love includes genuine concern – concern for your needs and well-being, and concern for your hopes and dreams.

★★★

It's true that, with God, everything is possible. Still, there are things that God cannot do. For instance, God cannot steal, cheat, or hate; because such flaws are foreign to Divine nature.

★★★

A miracle is anything that sparks a greater awareness of God's presence.

★★★

As you grow to trust that which cannot be seen or touched, a reassuring truth is revealed: Even when no one is within your sight or reach, you are not alone.

★★★

A SAMPLING OF PRAYERS

O Merciful God, I give you my worries. I release to you my fears and surrender to you my anxieties. Amen

O Loving God, allow me to receive your guidance, your patience, and your calmness. Help me to feel your loving presence. Amen

Surrounded by weakness, I ask for strength. Surrounded by pain, I ask for comfort. In the midst of confusion, I pray for clarity. And in the midst of sorrow, I pray for healing. Amen

In this time of chaos, I ask for a safe harbor. Ease my mind as you quiet the wind, and replenish my energy as you calm the sea. Give me the courage and resolve to carry on. Amen

Through your grace, O God, relieve my pain and quell my fear. Ease my suffering and lighten my burden. I ask to feel your heavenly comfort, your holy presence, and your Divine peace. Amen

O God, help me to understand your plan for me. Help me to fully know your will. Give me insight and discernment, so that I can distinguish the pathway from the detour, the real from the unreal, and the meaningful from the meaningless. Amen

May God bring you comfort and surround you with goodness and strength. May you be calmed and renewed. May you find wisdom and guidance on your journey, and may you come to know hope and joy. Amen

★★★

While there's a natural instinct to protect or shield your loved ones from pain, be mindful of what you pray for. Remember that life seldom unfolds in the way you expect. For example, what if your prayer for safety deprived a loved one from confronting a painful but transformative experience, something that would ultimately be helpful, healing, and enlightening? Such unforeseeable outcomes remind us that the most powerful prayers simply ask for God's will to be done. In truth, Divine plans are always better than human desires, even when our intentions are good. Through adversity, we are given an opportunity to grow in faith, patience, and trust. And through hardship, we are given a chance to learn what is true, and what is false; what is real, and what is illusion.

★★★

Does God really need a constant stream of human advice? Rather than automatically praying for a specific outcome, consider praying for the higher good.

★★★

Intentional living is an individual's purposeful attempt to live according to one's beliefs or values. This lifestyle choice is typically built on spiritual, moral, and ethical foundations or philosophies. Intentional living requires a mindful awareness of your core beliefs. Moreover, you must strive to act in a manner that genuinely reflects those core beliefs.

Intentional living embraces mindful and purposeful behavior in all circumstances. Reactional living, however, is making knee-jerk responses to people, situations, or events. What's more, such spontaneous responses are often contrary to one's core beliefs.

★★★

When it comes to comparing and judging, the ego's appetite is insatiable. Why does this person have more money? Or better health? Or a bigger house, and a newer car? Or a happier marriage, and an easier job? And why is this person more respected, or intelligent, or attractive? What about innocent babies born with shocking deformities? Why do young people die from tragic accidents? What about human bodies ravaged by disease? Why does the world have poverty and starvation? And why do horrible things happen to good people?

The ego's questions and grievances are endless. And if this one life on earth were, in truth, *all* that ever is or will be, then fits of jealousy and anger might be justified. Yet, an eternal afterlife holds the power to right all wrongs, to balance all scales, to heal all wounds, and to erase any misguided notions that life is unfair. Therein lies the mercy of God.

★★★

Regardless of the details, your problems are not unique. There are countless people around the world who are struggling with similar problems. You are not alone, nor have you been singled out for punishment. To regain clarity and calmness, try this Tibetan relaxation exercise ...

Breathe in – to yourself and all others – the kindness, compassion, and serenity needed to confront your challenges.

Breathe out your worry, fear, and suffering – and the worry, fear, and suffering of everyone in the world who is confronting similar challenges.

Repeat this deep, cleansing in-breath and out-breath as many times as you wish.

★★★

When something bad happens, perhaps you may ask, "Why me?" Yet, a more insightful question is, "Why not me?" But try to ask the question gently and compassionately.

★★★

Before you speak, ask if what you're about to say is true, kind, and helpful. If your words meet all three guidelines, then say them. If not, then silence is a better gift to offer.

★★★

We receive the life lessons we need. Frequently, they're not the ones we want.

★★★

Carol is a hospice caregiver. During her bedside visits, she observes pain and suffering. Because Carol cannot attach meaning or purpose to such suffering, she sees it as unfair. Moreover, she knows there are times when she's unable to mitigate a patient's pain. This realization triggers feelings of inadequacy. And as Carol starts doubting her abilities, guilt creeps in. Driving home from work, she notices a homeless man – a reminder of the suffering that's right in her own neighborhood. Again, Carol cannot find meaning or purpose to this man's pain – and she can't fix it. Later that evening, Carol watches the news on TV. She sees clear evidence of pain and suffering all across America and in nations around the world. And once more, she cannot find meaning to this widespread suffering, and she can't alleviate it. Carol wonders: *How could a God of mercy allow people to suffer?* Confused and dismayed, she starts to question God's existence. Unless Carol adopts a more realistic worldview – and embraces a more positive self-image – she could soon be trapped in a cycle of negative thoughts, such as: *The world is a mess, and God is nowhere to be found.* Or, *I'm not helping my patients. I'm letting everyone down.*

★★★

To believe that God is real is only the first part of your spiritual journey. Next, you must learn to trust your Creator. Right now, do you trust God enough to offer gratitude for *all* that happens, without exception? Those who understand Divine Order know that good ultimately triumphs over evil, and that life always prevails over death. This assurance removes all cause for worry or fear – and therein lies the grace of God.

★★★

People who don't believe in a benevolent God often have a difficult time reaching accurate conclusions about other matters as well. Such individuals are just too far removed from a reality-based foundation.

★★★

Perhaps you see evidence of Divinity while watching a beautiful sunset. But is God not equally visible as you witness a peaceful death?

★★★

Dressing a wound can be uncomfortable for the patient and unpleasant for the caregiver. Yet is this shared experience not an extension of God's mercy? Is there not an element of Divinity in many of your work-related tasks?

★★★

Advancing an agenda which contradicts Divine Order is similar to forcing a square peg into a round hole. Usually, it doesn't work very well.

★★★

Make spiritual work part of your routine. Try morning prayer, reflective reading, or meditation. Integrate art or music into your life, and add creative outlets such as writing, dancing, or performing.

★★★

Daily prayer, reflection, and meditation prepare you to receive God's gifts and blessings.

★★★

During periods of contemplative introspection, dare to stretch your comfort zone. Find the courage to explore the silent recesses of your mind, and find the resolve to discover the stillness deep within your heart. Travel light. Carry as little baggage as possible, and be filled with great hope and expectation.

★★★

Even when you've been traumatized, there is part of you that remains untouched and unaffected. The *awareness* of scars was never scarred.

★★★

Instead of having "thoughts" as your default mode, make "awareness" your new default mode.

★★★

First, close your eyes and focus on your breathing.

Next, allow your breathing to "cradle" your body.

Then, let go of your body.

Next, let go of time.

Then, let go of thoughts.

Next, focus on awareness.

Now, *be* the awareness.

★★★

After being shot, Gandhi expressed no anger, fear, or even surprise. He simply looked into the assassin's eyes; then, Gandhi folded his hands, repeated his mantra, and died. Decades of meditation had prepared him to accept, without judgment, the present moment, including the moment he left this world.

Meditation Mantra

I have enough

I do enough

I am enough

★★★

Gracious God, use me this day as an instrument of your will. Help me to be a conduit of your light, love, and peace.

Keep me safe this day, and protect me from evil and malice in all forms. Guide me through any obstacles that might prevent me from expressing the love that I am.

Allow me to feel your presence and experience your peace.

And for those who are hurting emotionally or spiritually – for those who are sick or dying – I send them my awareness, my love, and my willingness to be with them in spirit.

★★★

Believing requires faith, whereas knowing does not. For instance, if two people were conversing on an ocean shore, one might say, "I believe high tide will arrive tomorrow morning." But the other may reply, "I *know* high tide will arrive tomorrow at 8:15AM." This kind of supreme confidence might come from years of study and research, or it could be the byproduct of countless personal experiences. Either way, a journey was needed to arrive there. And so it is with one's perception of God. To conclude that there isn't a God actually requires no effort at all. But for those who are willing to dig deeper, to embark on an earnest search for truth, Divine grace will guide them to a more enlightened destination.

★★★

Closing reflection …

Do you believe there is a loving God? Why or why not? Do you *know* that God is real? If so, how have you reached this conclusion?

Are you in the process of building a personal relationship with God? If so, describe any changes in your life that might be tied to this effort.

Theologians suggest that the most powerful prayers are those which ask for God's will to be done. Why might this be true?

Spiritual teachers have written that trust solves all problems. What does this mean to you?

How might you nurture greater patience and grow more trusting of God?

★★★

DAY THIRTEEN

INTERCONNECTEDNESS

Each man and woman, in a self-determined tempo and with an individual voice, must discover and reaffirm the knowledge that all things are one thing, and that one thing is all things. *John Steinbeck*

★★★

Is fact stranger than fiction? Could a discussion of nature *vs.* nurture possibly explain how two lives unfold as though they are one? Perhaps you're a skeptic of destiny, or a cynic of coincidence. Nonetheless, prepare yourself for this amazing tale of the Jim twins.

University of Minnesota psychologist, Thomas Bouchard is best known for his research on the genetic influences found in identical twins who were separated at birth. Identical twins come from a single egg – fertilized by a single sperm – which splits shortly after the egg starts to develop. In 1979, Bouchard studied the "Jim twins" as they were called. In a test that measured personality types, their scores were so close that Bouchard noted, "It could have been the same person taking the test two times." He also learned that the Jim twins had nearly identical brain wave test results. And incredibly, the brothers had similar medical histories. But there's even more to the story.

Shortly after birth, the identical twin boys were adopted by different parents who happened to give their respective sons the name James. The boys grew up in Ohio and lived about fifty miles from one another. Still, they never met until Jim Lewis, at age thirty-seven, decided to track down his brother. Through court records, Jim Lewis located his twin, Jim Springer. They talked on the phone and agreed to meet one another for the very first time.

At their reunion, the Jim twins discovered they had much more in common than just their genes. Each had named his childhood dog "Toy." Both were married twice, first to women named Linda, and then to women named Betty. Each had a son named James Allen. Both were chain-smokers, enjoyed drinking beer, and had woodworking shops in their garages. Both drove Chevy trucks, and both worked as deputy sheriffs in the counties where they lived. Their remarkably similar journeys couldn't have been duplicated if the brothers had tried!

★★★

Nature offers convincing evidence of interconnectedness. Bees pollinate flowers and plants, including a variety of fruits, nuts, and vegetables – even as humans and animals are enjoying the honey produced by the bees. Ducks and geese, with help from their webbed feet, transfer fish eggs from one lake to the next, thereby increasing fish population and diversity. Humans have, throughout the ages, relied on animals for food and clothing. More recently, wildlife management strives to protect birds, animals, and fish from excessive harvesting. Of course, domesticated animals are cherished members of human families. Plants and insects, fish and fowl, animals and humans – all are joined and dependent on one another. Yet, this interconnectedness extends even further; for the animate and the inanimate share, on some level, a common bond – the same bond that ties the infinite to the infinitesimal.

★★★

In an interconnected universe, each person's spiritual growth contributes to the advancement and well-being of the greater whole.

★★★

People tend to embrace linear thinking, meaning that most of us perceive our world as an endless series of finite, straight lines. Additionally, each separate line starts and ends with an exact opposite. One line, for instance, begins with sweet and ends with bitter. Another starts with love and stops with hate. And yet another line begins with life and ends with death. However, linear thinking is misleading, primarily because people who focus on polarities tend to see an unruly, detached world rather than a beneficent, connected one. With this in mind, let's take a closer look at illusion *vs.* reality.

On earth, the western hemisphere's day blends seamlessly with the eastern hemisphere's night. Without fail, night's darkness slowly surrenders to the light of a new day. On our planet, north gradually joins with south, which meets again with north. And polar cold stretches to touch tropical heat, only to merge once more with numbing cold. Next, consider the seasons. Spring is an escort to summer; summer leads to autumn which heralds winter; and winter yields to another spring. Earth isn't a simple world made of separate lines. To the contrary, life is thriving in a complex network of interconnecting circles. This new vision is illuminating because, unlike lines, circles are perfect and unbroken. As it is with God, circles are the alpha and the omega, without beginning or end.

By embracing this shift in perception, you will see a more enduring, purposeful, and unified world. Then, it's easier to marvel at earth's wonder and beauty. It's easier to understand that, by design, life cannot be snuffed out; nor can the earth's splendor and abundance be erased by greed or jealousy, fear or hatred. From this new perspective, how could love have an opposite? Moreover, how could God's children be anything but brothers and sisters? For indeed, love is an everlasting circle. Love is a sacred, universal bond which cannot be broken by a tragic accident, a brutal crime, a painful disease, or an untimely death. Of course life, too, has no opposite. For in the circle of life, each ending is but a new beginning. And each new beginning holds promise beyond what you can imagine.

★★★

Artists, poets, and healers have long paid tribute to humanity's connection with nature ...

"Surely there was profound comfort within the cliff homes, for their stature, their vision, and their safety against the mother rock. Families must have snuggled together as torrents of rain came down like silver curtains, and as wolfish winds howled and clawed at the mountain." Mary Austin, 1924

"Every granite mesa is mirrored by a motionless cloud mesa, no matter how hot the day or how blue the sky. Such immense tables of rock cannot be without the attendant clouds which are a part of them – as smoke is of the fire, or foam is of the wave." Willa Cather, 1927

"In the hour of the desert's gray splendor, it is good to be among the dunes. Across their spherical curves, sharp shadows grow long. In the mystery of twilight, softness veils the desolation, and coolness comes with a velvet touch. Though all reflections have gone, the western sky remains aglow in luminous pink and lavender." Ross Calvin, 1948

"The Grand Canyon is a living, pulsating, ever-changing being. From walls of brown and black, scarlet flames stretch outward, then dissolve among streaks of orange and purple. Around its domes and arches and spires, a soul dwells. And in its deepest recess, its innermost gorge, is the very spirit of our living God." R. B. Stanton, 1909

I stood alone, gazing upon the Sangre de Cristo Mountains. A singular rock formation had captured my interest. Suddenly a deep voice, vibrant with emotion, pierced the silence: "Do you not think that all life comes from the mountain?" I turned and saw an Indian elder – moccasins had helped him approach undetected. Reflecting on his heaven-knows-how-far-reaching question, I thought, *Of course all life comes from the mountain; nothing could be more obvious.* So I replied, "Everyone can see that you speak the truth." Carl Jung, 1925

★★★

Swiss psychiatrist Carl Jung received worldwide acclaim for his contributions to psychoanalysis, anthropology, philosophy, and religious studies. In the following quotations by Jung, try reading "between the lines." Can you find hints of interconnectedness?

A fixation on thinking is usually accompanied by a feeling of inferiority.

The art of living is the most distinguished and rarest of all the arts.

A directed life is better, richer, and healthier than an aimless one.

Death is only a transition – one part of a life-process. In this respect, death is a goal to which one can strive.

Humans share a collective unconscious; and from it, consciousness has developed.

A great work of art rises far above the artist's personal life; it is born of the heart and spirit.

Religious convictions are often treated like Sunday attire: They are tried, then set aside like worn-out clothes.

The human being who suffers has not yet discovered life's meaning.

In order to live well, all that's needed is faith, hope, love, and insight.

Happiness would lose its meaning if it were not balanced by sadness.

You cannot change anything until you accept it.

You are what you do, not what you say you'll do.

I am not what has happened to me, I am what I choose to become.

Those who look outward will dream; those who look inward will awaken.

First, understand why other people irritate you. Then, you will gain an understanding of yourself.

In chaos, there is a cosmos; in disorder, a secret order.

There is no growth without pain.

The purpose of human existence is to kindle a light of meaning in the darkness of mere being.

★★★

Every disaster, be it natural or man-made, brings an opportunity to serve and advance the greater good. Each episode of upheaval offers a transformational opportunity to achieve oneness and wholeness. And herein rests the grace of God.

★★★

In life, as in nature, there is a time and a season for everything under heaven. And because change is inevitable, some seasons will be smoother, easier, and perhaps happier than others. Often, these changing seasons are beyond your control. Yet, while you may not be able to control what happens, you *can* control your perception of what happens. By the way, if you're searching for stability, for that which is steadfast and everlasting, turn to God: Divine love is timeless and changeless.

★★★

In a perfect world, every human interaction would include an exchange of gifts. And yes, many of our common interactions already achieve this goal. If your dog is sick, a veterinarian offers a gift of treatment in return for the gift of money. Or if you're lost and ask a stranger for directions, his gift of guidance is matched by your gifts of a warm smile and a heartfelt, *Thank you!* And there are opportunities to be creative as well. For example, a farmer could plant corn on his neighbor's field and – as payment – the landowner could receive a portion of the crop. Or a carpenter might build a new garage for a plumber who, in exchange, might remodel a bathroom in the carpenter's home. The goal is straightforward: Make sure that your exchanges and interactions with others aren't too one-sided.

In terms of care giving, what gifts do you offer? What gifts do you receive? In truth, joyful giving and grateful receiving are gifts of equal value. Are you sometimes discouraged by rude or grumpy patients who don't appreciate your gift of service? If so, how do you overcome such feelings? On the other hand, can you recall patient visits where, after leaving, you felt as though you had received more than you had given?

★★★

Closing Reflection ...

Overall, do you feel that the "gift exchanges" between you and your patients are equitable and reasonably balanced? If not, what can you do differently?

★★★

Walking in a winter woods: hauntingly beautiful, reverently silent, wonderfully still. Faithful trails serving humans and animals alike. First, a sheltered valley. Next, a weathered ridge-top. Footprints dotting a blanket of snow: virgin and holy, healing and affirming, refreshing and renewing. Moving forward: skeletal starkness, unabashed nakedness, dancing sunlight, twinkling ice. Mother Nature knows nothing of yesterdays or tomorrows. Leafless limbs pointing the way. Uphill, then down. Flat, then rocky. Moving forward: careful steps, quiet thoughts, crooked smile. Observing. Greeting what *is*.

★★★

DAY FOURTEEN

BYRON KATIE

Everything happens *for* you, not to you. You don't have
to like it, but it's easier if you do. *Byron Katie*

★★★

Born in Texas and raised in California, Byron Katie was a quiet, thoughtful little girl. She grew to be smart, attractive, energetic, and talented. Katie married her high school sweetheart, Robert. Together, they started a real estate company that thrived and, rather quickly, made them wealthy and respected. Katie and Robert built a grand riverfront house and hosted lavish parties. They had all the trappings of success. But for Katie, it wasn't enough. Nothing could please or satisfy her for long. Katie's search for happiness through money and status left her increasingly frustrated. By having everything, yet seeking more, she never had a moment of contentment.

Katie's choices eventually led to alcohol abuse, narcotic addiction, and clinical depression. She divorced Robert, and quickly remarried – this time to Paul, a friend fifteen years her senior. Though Paul was kind and attentive, Katie's self-loathing and destructive behavior continued. Later, she described it this way: "I spent my days in bed, usually drinking, smoking, ranting, popping pills, and eating ice cream. I weighed over two hundred pounds. Nothing felt good; nothing brought peace. I was obese, but starving. I was medicated, but couldn't relieve the pain. I was dead, but still breathing."

Paul drove Katie, now forty-three years old, to a halfway house. There, she chose to live in the attic and sleep on the floor. One day, while roaming on her hands and knees, Katie spotted a bug. She examined this creature closely, but didn't touch it. Then she gazed into its beady eyes for what seemed like hours. As time passed, Katie began to feel a kinship with this bug. They were, after all, on the same planet within a vast universe. They were actually sharing the floor of the very same room. And somehow, both were products of the same Creator. She mused, *What an unlikely set of circumstances.* It finally dawned on her that all life forms are interconnected, perhaps even dependent on one another. This revelation prompted a question: Do these complex relationships include, by design, an element of responsibility, an incumbent duty of stewardship? She thought, *Of course they do!* And this insightful realization brought new meaning to Katie's life – meaning she had long been searching for. Instantly, the bug was beautiful! Every living thing was beautiful, and life was exactly how God intended it to be!

With renewed vigor and determination, Katie emerged from her valley of despair. She grew closer to God and, aided by an improved way to see the world, found lasting inner peace. In truth, Katie was born again; her life was forever changed. Therapists periodically hear amazing stories from people who were transformed by an unexpected "ah-ha" moment. It's never known if, or when, such epiphanies might occur. But it's reasonable to presume that these seminal events are, by their nature, Divine.

Here's how Katie recalls her personal transformation:

"It was as though I had awakened from an ancient dream. Everything I looked at glowed with radiance. I was in a state of childlike awe, and there was only love. I was drenched with love, wild with love, blissful with love. Then I saw the image of an old woman. She wore a paisley dress, and her hair was styled in a bun. She was angelic, gracious, and wise. Through her, I came to realize that I didn't have to suffer, that there's never a need to suffer. I knew that life unfolds perfectly. We always receive exactly what we need. God is everywhere and part of everything. Just embrace life. Trust it and love it unconditionally. The angel lady visited me from time to time, always wearing the same frumpy dress. I'm not sure if she was real or not, but I felt her outpouring of love, and I cherished her guidance."

Adapted from an article by Daniel Millman

★★★

Heavenly angels can reach out to people by appearing in their dreams as visions and voices. Angels might offer comfort, guidance, assurance, or helpful insights. They may also appear in human form to interact or converse with someone for a brief time. In either case, angels are God's messengers.

★★★

Byron Katie developed a clever technique to examine her own thoughts. She calls it "the work" and this innovative method can help you break free from stressful thinking patterns. You start by answering four questions. *Is the thought true? Are you absolutely sure that it's true? How are you reacting to this thought?* And then, *Who would you be without this thought?* The next step is what Katie calls "the turnaround." You repeat the original, negative thought in an opposing view. Finally, you list three reasons why this "turnaround thought" might be true. Here's an example.

Jane is a hospice nurse on her way to visit a home care patient, Mr. Jones for a second time. During last week's initial visit, Mr. Jones was angry, combative, and disrespectful. Jane thought, *This visit will be unbearable!* She started feeling anxious and stressed while pulling into the patient's driveway. But let's re-examine Jane's original thought, as suggested by Katie's method.

- **Was her thought true?** Perhaps.
- **Was Jane absolutely sure it was true?** Not really.
- **How was Jane reacting to her thought?** She felt anxious and stressed.
- **Who would Jane be without this thought?** She would still be a nurse getting ready to visit a patient, but she would be more calm and relaxed.

Now for the turnaround ...

Jane's original thought – *This visit will be unbearable!* – is replaced by the opposite outcome: *This will be a wonderful visit!* Followed by: *And I can list three reasons why.*

First: Mr. Jones needs my help, and I chose to be a nurse so I could help others. It gives my life meaning, and I feel good about that.

Second: During my previous visit, Mr. Jones said his pain was an 8 out of 10. With new meds in place, it's likely he will be more comfortable and, therefore, more pleasant.

Third: When my interventions alleviate a patient's suffering, I know in my heart that I've done my best. I don't always need to receive praise.

So if you were Jane, would you change your mind about that negative thought? Would you choose to let it go and allow the stress and anxiety to go with it?

Byron Katie: Thoughts and reflections ...

I discovered that when I believed my fearful thoughts, I suffered. But when I realized that my thoughts were often misguided, I felt much better. I learned that, sometimes, suffering is optional, and it was a liberating insight.

Nothing happens ahead of its time, and what needs to happen always happens. Whenever you oppose what *is* happening, you're going to experience anxiety. You're going to feel a sense of separation from reality.

Peace is found on the inside. Where have you been looking?

Being kind to oneself is good medicine.

A thought is harmless, unless you believe it.

Suffering is a signal that you're confused, that you're believing a lie.

It's not your job to like me; it's mine!

Reality is always kinder than your thinking.

When we start to get honest with ourselves, the space between our thoughts grows wider and wider.

Ask yourself, *Is this happening?* If the answer is yes, then it's supposed to be happening.

Death comes in its own sweet way. Until you know that death is as good as life, you're going to assume the role of God – and death will always hurt.

★★★

Closing reflection ...

No one walks alone when crossing the bridge to eternity. And this world's beauty falls far short of what awaits you as the pathway vanishes and time ends with it. *ACIM*

★★★

Crossing the Bar

Sunset first, then evening star
And one sweet call for me!
There shall be no moaning of the bar
When I put out to sea.

The moving tides that never sleep
Bear crests of sound and foam.
And the Maker of this boundless deep
Will guide me safely home.

Twilight first, then nighttime bell
And after that the dawn!
There shall be no wailing of farewell
When I at last am gone.

While on my trip of time and place
The waves will take me far.
And I hope to see my Pilot's face
When I have crossed the bar.

Adapted from the poem by Lord Alfred Tennyson

★★★

DAY FIFTEEN

GRATEFULNESS

Gratitude makes sense of our past, brings peace for today,
and creates vision for tomorrow. *Melody Beattie*

★★★

With the potential to promote dramatic and lasting positive effects, mental health experts agree that gratitude is one of life's most vitalizing ingredients. Clinical research has shown that expressions of gratitude reduce the risk for depression, anxiety, and substance abuse disorders. Whether it stems from the acceptance of someone's kindness, an appreciation for majesty and beauty, or the recognition of gifts and blessings in one's own life, gratitude enhances virtually every aspect of the human experience. Some of our most cherished moments are those in which we receive love that's been freely and generously given. Indeed, much of life's significance pertains to giving and receiving gifts – an affirmation of life's inherent goodness.

True gratitude is the antithesis of being focused on oneself. Those who are grateful recognize that they have been blessed by the grace of others. Therefore, the ultimate goal is to find creative ways to pass that grace forward, to find opportunities to bless the lives of others. Gratitude is a universal human attribute that's found in virtually all people, of all cultures, worldwide. It's tied to the wonder and awe that emerge from an interconnected humanity. Indeed, gratitude is woven into the very fabric of human nature.

Studies indicate that grateful people are more likely to agree with statements such as: *It's important to appreciate each day that I'm alive* and, *I know my life is easier because of other people's efforts* or, *For me, life is much more of a gift than a burden.* Gratitude is a sustainable approach to life that isn't dependent on an individual's circumstances. Still, it involves a conscious choice and requires mindful cultivation. People who practice gratitude set aside time to reflect on life's little pleasures. They often see life events and personal encounters as blessings. They take the time to write and send thank-you notes, and they make regular entries in their gratitude journals.

Gratitude practice includes an awareness of what is going right in one's life, and it recognizes the contributions that others are making. Those who are practicing gratitude shift their attention from the negative to the positive. Additionally, gratitude practice includes an acknowledgment that difficult and painful experiences serve as teachable moments. Those who reach a high level of gratefulness are able to heal from past wounds and look to the future with vigor, enthusiasm, and optimism. Moreover, surprising changes may occur: a relationship that was once taken for granted might become more valued; a different perspective on life's meaning and purpose could emerge; or a sudden epiphany may lead to new insights on truth and reality.

★★★

More on gratitude ...

- Gratitude can be either a fleeting emotion, or a long-term feeling that becomes part of someone's personality.
- People who often feel and express gratitude tend to be happier, even when their life circumstances are more challenging.
- Gratitude relieves the symptoms of stress and depression.
- Gratitude fosters greater empathy.
- Those who frequently express gratitude feel less lonely and isolated.
- Gratitude promotes a greater sense of well-being and an improved quality of life.
- Expressions of gratitude lead to closer, more meaningful and committed relationships.
- Gracious people tend to express gratitude even for small things.
- Family, friends, coworkers, love, kindness, opportunities, careers, beauty, abundance, gifts, fields, flowers, woodlands, birds, animals, mountains, oceans, food, clothing, shelter, art,

music, and Divinity. There is literally no end to what you can be thankful for.

★★★

Everyone shares a common purpose in life: to grow in love and faith.

★★★

Faith makes things possible, not easy. Yet, as you become more spiritually mature, day-to-day challenges are less daunting. Then, life *does* get easier.

★★★

A positive worldview nurtures a healthy perception of self, and promotes a sense of well-being. One way to keep a positive attitude is to focus on abundance, rather than lack. Depending on where and when you look, nature offers endless reminders of abundance: water, soil, plants, sunlight, trees, birds, animals, flowers, clouds, stars, and so on.

★★★

From the ego's perspective, you never have enough – enough love, appreciation, money, or possessions. Or maybe you think you're lacking in talent, fame, status, beauty, or intelligence. Yet, could it be that "not enough" is just a misguided perception? Are peace and happiness tied to having enough?

★★★

Spiritual teachers suggest that, at birth, you've already been given what you truly need.

★★★

On a primal level, Abraham Maslow concluded ...

If there's no air to breathe, you won't be worried about having water to drink.

If there's no water to drink, you won't be worried about having food to eat.

If there's no food to eat, you won't be worried about having long-term shelter.

If there's no long-term shelter, you won't be worried about pursuing a career, finding a relationship, or exploring metaphysics.

★★★

Hope *vs.* Gratitude

Hope and gratitude are both important to your mental stability and well-being. Yet, they are not of equal value. Hope is founded on a future desire that may, or may not materialize, whereas gratitude is linked to something that's meaningful to you now. Gratitude, therefore, holds greater power to heal, uplift, and inspire. Moreover, by expressing thankfulness, you're making a conscious choice to focus on the positive. You're appreciating what you already have, instead of wanting something you don't have.

Power *vs.* Force

Profound contrasts distinguish power from force. First and foremost, God is a Higher Power. Therefore, power is a derivative of love, whereas force is a product of fear. While force may win short-term gains, love never fails – meaning that power triumphs in the end. Power liberates, uplifts, and inspires, while force enslaves, controls, and manipulates. Oppression and exploitation are man-made constructs that are destined to wither. Indeed, whatever is upheld by force will eventually collapse.

Human hearts are the wellspring of power, whereas force is ego-driven. Your ego seeks authority and glory, while your heart yearns for righteousness and humility. Your ego is angry, envious, and self-absorbed, but your heart is kind, patient, and selfless. Your ego prefers to judge and punish, while your heart wishes to serve and comfort. Ultimately, this is why you must choose to follow your heart.

★★★

Holding a position of authority, or possessing great wealth – such circumstances are inherently neutral, neither good nor evil. What matters is how they are used. Authority can either help, or hinder; and wealth can either liberate, or oppress.

★★★

The next time you go to a supermarket, be aware of how many shelves there are. Then take note of the wide variety of foods and products. Notice how each shelf is overflowing with desirable items that you may wish to buy. In the produce department, notice how the colorful, delicious fruits and vegetables are displayed. Imagine how they were carefully nurtured and harvested, and how they were intentionally shipped to a local market for you to purchase and enjoy.

And when you shop at a department store, notice how many items have been assembled for you, a valued customer, to examine: shoes and socks, coats and hats, shirts and jeans, vacuum cleaners and hair dryers, toaster ovens and coffee makers, televisions, computers, and so on. Are such examples of abundance not deserving of your awareness and gratitude?

★★★

Giving thanks helps us grow closer to God. Gratefulness reminds us that we are dependent on Divine gifts and blessings.

★★★

Create a gratitude journal

There are many ways to start journaling and, depending on your preference, there are a number of options as to how often you write. Some people like to write a short time each day, while others choose to write a longer time once a week. Frequently, people settle on a routine that's somewhere in between. In any case, journaling should be a heartfelt commitment. Studies show that gratitude journaling promotes healthy physiological changes in brain chemistry. It nurtures positive neural networking and improves life balance. Simply stated, gratitude journaling gently guides you away from negative thought patterns.

If you wish, you can start by journaling some of your earliest memories. What are the greatest gifts and blessings you remember? Describe your favorite times with grandparents, aunts, uncles, cousins, neighbors, and friends. Have you been helped by a favorite teacher, a generous neighbor, or a kind stranger? Write about your fondest memories with your mom or dad. While growing up, what were some of the fun things you did with siblings or close friends? Make sure to include special occasions, vacations, and holidays as you move through the years. Have you received any gifts or blessings from God? Are you grateful for aspects of your health? Have you ever gained wisdom or courage by overcoming adversity?

Moving closer to the present, are you receiving gifts from a spouse? Are you grateful for children, grandchildren, or close friends? Are you blessed by your hospice career, and your relationships with patients and coworkers? Write about materialistic blessings, favorite hobbies, and volunteer activities? Do you see beauty and goodness in the world? Do you meet kind and thoughtful people? Do you find evidence of love and abundance around you? Are there spiritual or intangible blessings to include in your journal? Has someone offered you forgiveness? Are blessings and joys sometimes disguised as simple, even trivial moments of everyday life?

Once you are journaling in real time, you could choose to write down three blessings every day. Or another option is to write about what went right in your day, and also *why* it was right. This approach strengthens brain circuitry for positive emotions and thoughts, while also establishing a desired cause and effect connection. In other words, you are preparing yourself to see more positives in the world by cementing the memory of a positive event. And when you write things down, you're using your brain to make those thoughts strong and lasting.

★★★

Closing reflection ...

Take a moment to examine the difference between your needs and your desires.

★★★

Look at your life, both past and present. What are you most grateful for? Offer praise for your most cherished blessings. Celebrate them!

★★★

DAY SIXTEEN

HEALTH AND WELL-BEING, PART ONE

Health is real wealth, not pieces of gold and silver. *Gandhi*

★★★

In general, ethics guide your workplace choices and behavior, while morals guide your personal choices and behavior. Right and wrong are extensions of your core beliefs, and your choices are manifestations of free will.

Though it's wise to limit your judgment of others, there *is* a difference between right and wrong. There *is* a difference between a helpful and a harmful choice. And there *is* a difference between appropriate and inappropriate behavior. Sometimes the lines are blurred. But in terms of *your* life and *your* decisions, remember: Maintaining high ethical and moral standards is always a good choice.

Have you fallen into the trap of thinking Choice A is the moral equivalent of Choice B?

Are you following your moral compass when choosing what you watch, what you listen to, and who you spend time with?

By listening to your heart, you're more likely to make virtuous choices.

Before saying or doing something you may regret, ask yourself: *Will my words and actions be expressions of love?*

★★★

It's a healthy choice to take breaks from reading, watching, and listening to the news. Much of the content is disturbing and discouraging. Often, the reporting is agenda-driven. Yet, regardless of the circumstances, constant exposure to negativity is disheartening. It sours your mood and taints your worldview.

★★★

Love is alive and well, despite what the news may report. For instance, you might see the devastating effects of a hurricane or an earthquake. You might hear details about the loss of life and property. Yet, there's normally a huge outpouring of aid following a natural disaster, and rarely do you see news coverage for these gestures of kindness.

★★★

Over one thousand studies have shown that children and adolescents exposed to violent movies and video games exhibit more aggressive, violent behavior than normal.

★★★

We've not yet unraveled the sublime mysteries of sleep. However, one thing is known for sure: Sleep deprivation causes chronic fatigue. A lack of sleep may eventually lead to more serious health problems or, in rare cases, death. Nearly everyone endures an occasional restless night. We toss and turn and simply cannot fall asleep. And when we finally doze for a bit, we're trapped in a dream cycle. We awaken – and feel exhausted. In order to feel rested and energized in the morning, we must have a period of deep sleep, a time when the mind is completely free of thoughts and dreams. Just as there's a spiritual side to wakefulness, our sleeping hours have a spiritual dimension as well. In that realm of absolute silence and stillness, we unconsciously connect with God. We join with an infinite, Divine presence. In truth, it's a time of healing, a time to experience heavenly peace as we once knew it. Then, we awaken refreshed and renewed.

★★★

Fatigue makes us confront enemies that were vanquished long ago.

★★★

When you're unable to fall asleep, try counting your blessings. Go back to your earliest childhood memories. Identify the people who were loving and helpful. Reflect on the blessings you received as a child. Next, move on to your years as a teenager; and then, as a young adult. Relax your body. Express gratitude for the gifts that have shaped your life. Continue counting your blessings until you gently drift off to sleep.

★★★

In deep sleep, we connect with the Divine. In silence and stillness, we join with our Creator. These holy moments are healing and restorative. Indeed, we cannot live without them.

★★★

For your much needed rest and renewal, try to set aside some unstructured time each day.

★★★

A small, indoor water feature will add the soothing, peaceful sound of flowing water to an office space or a room in your home.

★★★

When repressed, anger is toxic. However, if venting anger becomes habitual and routine, then one must identify its source, bless it, and let it go.

★★★

You don't have to escape to the country in order to unwind. Urban settings also offer renewal opportunities. For example, a park bench overlooking a fountain, a basketball court, or a children's playground.

★★★

When feeling tired or run down, the last thing you may want to do is exercise. Yet, a vigorous workout is a great way to rejuvenate your body and mind. Do you see the paradox? Sometimes you gain energy by expending it!

★★★

A prolonged and uncharacteristic shortage of patience and tolerance is a sure sign of burnout. Other indicators include profound fatigue, a change in eating or sleeping habits, lingering pessimism, a flat affect, a decrease in job satisfaction, or an increase in absenteeism.

★★★

If you find yourself worrying to the point where it's affecting your performance at work, your enjoyment at home, or your ability to get a good night's sleep ...

1. Try setting aside one, ten minute block of time each day that is dedicated entirely to: Worrying! During this daily routine, it's okay to worry about anything you wish – without feeling guilty.
2. Of course, there's a follow-up responsibility as well. You are not permitted to worry during any other time of that 24 hour period. So be aware of your thoughts; and when you catch yourself worrying, let go of all negativity and say, *I will not worry about anything until tomorrow!*

★★★

Not-doing allows life to unfold at its own pace. It's a deliberate choice to invoke patience and *not* try to force or manipulate what *is*. Plus, there's a surprising benefit: not-doing can empower you to be more effective and productive than ever.

★★★

Not-doing requires discipline. Moreover, such discipline is reinforced by an understanding that real benefits are gained by making this choice.

★★★

Not-doing is a way to simplify life and identify what is important and meaningful. Simplicity keeps you from feeling overwhelmed. In order to simplify, you might need to say "no" to those who ask for more.

When you feel overextended – when there are too many demands on your time – strive to keep things simple.

★★★

Someone who's not-doing is different from a do-nothing. Not-doing doesn't mean that you're ignoring responsibilities or obligations.

★★★

Are you ready to challenge your mind? Try to think of three different scenarios in which you can say something without talking, go somewhere without traveling, or gain something without doing.

★★★

Looking at your watch, you might say, "Oh my, it's *now* again. It just keeps happening over and over!"

★★★

When you live one day at a time, each morning is a fresh start – a new opportunity to make healthy, life-affirming choices!

★★★

Try this mindfulness exercise ...

Make a deliberate choice to do certain activities in slow motion, things like brushing your teeth, getting dressed, preparing a meal, or doing the dishes. If you reduce your normal speed by 50%, these routine tasks may become more interesting and enjoyable. Moreover, this slow-motion technique can help you stay more grounded in the present moment.

★★★

Reminisce the past, but don't be obsessed with it. Don't live there!

★★★

Don't get flustered by the relentless drama of this world — and don't be disheartened by the pervasive negativity tied to it.

★★★

Compassion fatigue leads to emotional withdrawal. As a result, compassion fatigue not only denies your patients the empathy they deserve, it steals those moments of pride and joy you would otherwise receive from your work. What's more, emotional withdrawal strains your relationships with friends and family members.

★★★

High achievers frequently establish unrealistically high standards for themselves — standards which they cannot meet. Next, these same high achievers will judge themselves based on how they think others are evaluating them, even though such assumptions are often wrong. The inevitable conclusion is: They are letting others down.

★★★

When you're hurting emotionally or spiritually, examine and acknowledge your feelings. Then, allow compassion to surround your pain. Be as kind to yourself as you are to a patient or loved one.

★★★

It isn't a sign of weakness to ask for help. Asking for help is not only an act of self-compassion, it can also be a gift to others.

★★★

We often confuse our thoughts with something entirely different: reality.

★★★

Thoughts are usually harmless unless you take them personally. Then, they can be devastating. For example, thoughts like: *I'm stupid. I'm unworthy.*

★★★

Toni Bernhard, a lawyer and author who has endured chronic pain for over thirty years, points out that living in the present moment doesn't necessarily shelter you from suffering. In fact, unfolding events or situations always hold the potential to be painful. Yet, as Bernhard teaches, you can be accepting of what *is*, and your acceptance can include calmness and compassion. In addition to predictable physiological changes, pain stimulates emotional responses such as fear, anger, and frustration. And soon thereafter, your mind will create a story about the pain, something like: *It isn't fair. This pain will never go away. Why me?*

Here's the message to remember. While you may not be able to change how your body reacts to pain, you do have the ability to reshape your perceptions of painful moments. In addition, you can write a more truthful story, perhaps something like: *This, too, shall pass.* Thought patterns, whether negative or positive, become habitual. So the most effective response for pain is calm acceptance, not fearful resistance. For instance, someone with a history of migraines typically experiences the same physical and visual sensations just prior to an episode of excruciating pain. A resistant, fearful reaction to those familiar sensations might be: *Oh, no! I can't stand another headache right now!* A more truthful, accepting response would be: *I've endured migraine pain before. I know I can do it again.*

★★★

Negative self-talk frequently stems from an unconscious belief that you should be someone other than who – or what – you are. As a result, there's an underlying disappointment and discomfort with your perception of self. With that in mind, try this two-step intervention. First, acknowledge that you – like everyone else – will always make innocent mistakes. Second, understand that your choices will not meet everyone's expectations or approval.

★★★

Examples of negative self-talk include: *No one understands or appreciates me. This is the worst ever! I'm all alone. Why is God punishing me? I don't deserve to be happy. This misery will never end!*

★★★

Remind yourself of the impermanent nature of pain. Recognize that God is the source of grace and mercy. And remember that God will never forsake or abandon you.

★★★

While moods and emotions are short-lived, feelings of victimization, unworthiness, guilt, and shame can last a lifetime.

★★★

The impermanence in our lives – relationships, jobs, health, finances, housing, and so on – contributes to an environment of uncertainty. Spiritual teachers proclaim that bliss is found where peace and change coexist. Because uncertainty is an inevitable part of the human condition, the quality of your life will improve dramatically if you can find a way to be at peace with change.

When you awaken in the morning, reflect on how you cannot possibly know what the day will bring. Yet, welcome it nonetheless. Embrace it, and give it all the attention and passion you can summon.

★★★

The flowerless bush is perfect. As a rosebud forms, the bush is perfect. As the rosebud blooms, the bush is perfect. As the blossom withers, the bush is perfect. And as the withered blossom drops to the ground, the flowerless bush is perfect.

★★★

Take a close look at these ten, stress-relieving tips ...

1. Instead of relying on your memory, make a list of your daily appointments and things to do.
2. Most of what you want are preferences, not needs. Don't obsess over preferences.
3. Simplify, simplify, simplify.
4. Before facing a stressful obligation, visualize how confident and successful you will be.
5. If you're struggling with a problem, seek advice from someone you admire and trust.
6. Focus on being understanding, rather than being understood.
7. Stop that negative self-talk!
8. Do the unpleasant tasks first, then enjoy the rest of your day.
9. Concentrate on one thing at a time. That way, you will always be doing your best.
10. Be willing to forgive. Accept that you live in an imperfect world.

★★★

A diamond is just a piece of charcoal that handled stress exceptionally well.

★★★

Soak in a hot bath and light a scented candle for added relaxation. Calm water, a flickering flame, and a comforting fragrance promote equanimity.

★★★

Try these seven ways to enrich your life ...

1. Be honest with yourself.
2. Look in a mirror and say, *I love you just the way you are!*
3. Be willing to forgive yourself. After all, mistakes are your best teachers.
4. When you receive a compliment, let it settle into the depths of your soul.
5. Apologize when you're wrong, and don't keep score.
6. Laugh, laugh, and laugh some more.
7. Remind people how much you love them.

★★★

Are you looking for a quick and easy way to be more positive?

Instead of saying, *I have to ...*

Try saying, *I get to ...*

I get to go shopping and buy things that I like.

I get to do the laundry and have clean clothes to wear.

I get to drive 12 hours and visit my best friend.

This technique is called reframing, and it puts a positive spin on something that otherwise might be viewed as a burden or chore.

★★★

As a caregiver, you can reframe a catastrophe – change your initial perception – to something more positive.

★★★

In heaven, you get to read holy books for all of eternity. In hell, you have to read holy books for all of eternity. See, perception *does* make a difference!

★★★

Some of our most life-threatening health problems can be linked specifically to drug and alcohol abuse. Desperate to escape what seems to be unbearable pain, more and more men, women, and teens are abusing both illicit and prescribed drugs. A significant percentage of abusers become drug dependent and, eventually, develop a full-blown addiction disorder.

Addicts are determined to obtain their desired drug, regardless of the harm they may cause to others or themselves in the procurement effort. Addiction also drives people to act irrationally when the addictive substance is absent from their central nervous system. Therefore, addicts seldom make responsible choices or enjoy healthy relationships. And because addictions can trigger abusive behavior, addicts hold the potential to harm nearly everyone they encounter.

Human beings are able to experience physical, emotional, and spiritual pain. So it makes sense that a mix of physical, psychological, and spiritual interventions are typically used to treat the destructive forces of addiction. Relapses are common. But there are breakthroughs, too – moments of clarity when people realize that they want to be clean and sober more than anything else. Then, through holistic therapy and hard work, long-term sobriety is attainable.

★★★

Reaching out to a Higher Power – acknowledging that we need God's assistance – keeps us humble. And humility helps tame our ego, a vital step in staying clean and sober.

★★★

In a misguided effort to demonstrate superiority, someone consumed by anger, hate, and rage might — with little or no provocation — verbally or physically attack an innocent family member, friend, or even a total stranger. The aggressive behavior may be a projection of the attacker's self-loathing, which can stem from unconscious feelings such as inferiority, guilt, shame, and unworthiness.

When examining abnormal aggression more closely, one might ask, *Why does this person have hidden feelings of inferiority, guilt, shame, or unworthiness?* Possible answers include:

- The person was verbally and/or physically abused as a child.
- The person was abandoned by a parent, or both parents.
- The person has not discovered a healthy meaning or purpose to life.

These same issues — abuse, abandonment, and meaninglessness — can lead to clinical depression. And in extreme cases, they culminate in self-inflicted harm.

★★★

Here's a suggestion for the next time you tweak a shoulder, sprain a knee, or twist an ankle ...

Immediately following an injury, place one hand (or both hands) directly on top of the source of your pain. Close your eyes and silently reach out to God. Ask for healing. In your mind, create a picture of Divine light surrounding your injury. Then, envision God's light penetrating, soothing, and healing the injured area. Keep your eyes closed and your hand (or hands) touching the source of the pain. Continue to create these visions of healing for five to ten minutes. End by whispering, *Thank you.*

Even if you ultimately require medical attention, this spiritual intervention can significantly accelerate your healing.

★★★

Closing reflection ...

What are the most rewarding aspects of your work as a hospice caregiver?

Regarding the self-care tips offered in this chapter, what changes can you make right now to improve your life at work and at home?

Do you believe effective self-care holds the potential to extend your hospice career? Why or why not?

★★★

DAY SEVENTEEN

HEALTH AND WELL-BEING, PART TWO

> Your life is like a bank account. Good choices
> are good investments. *Bethenny Frankel*

★★★

There's a good chance that you're interacting with teammates who think they can remain healthy and resilient simply by being stoic. That's a fallacy – and here's the truth: As a caregiver, you *will* experience pain. It's inevitable and inescapable. That's why it's important to learn how to endure pain and mitigate suffering. By definition, pain is neurological. Suffering, however, is the meaning you attach to pain. It's a perception, whether conscious or unconscious.

Physical pain produces neurological and physiological changes. Immediately, your brain releases adrenaline in preparation for a "fight or flight" response. At the same time, pain elevates your heart rate and blood pressure. In addition, pain may cause hyperventilation or spark anxiety and panic. Finally, pain creates muscle tension and triggers the release of cortisol, a steroid produced by the adrenal gland. These dramatic changes – if they occur frequently – have an incredibly negative impact on your health. In this altered state, you can't think clearly or communicate effectively. You may, in fact, be unable to competently perform even basic care giving tasks.

Understand that long-term emotional and spiritual pain can damage your health just as much as physical pain. Though commonly overlooked, emotional and spiritual pain lead to chronic stress and, ultimately, have devastating effects on the human body. The longer you stay in a state of stress, the more function you lose: discernment, cognitive skills, communication skills, and motor skills. Your level of compassion drops. You start to withdraw from those you love, and your thoughts become more negative. Eventually, stressors may lead to digestive system disorders or even fertility problems. And of course, you're more likely to make mistakes when stressed.

Take a moment to review these additional insights on pain and care giving ...

Primary trauma is something that happens to you personally. You only have to experience one event to have PTSD symptoms.

Secondary trauma is witnessing another person's trauma, or listening to stories of trauma. Typically, you would experience multiple events before having PTSD symptoms.

Resistance is the hidden culprit in pain-triggered events. By choosing to accept pain, rather than resist it, you can lessen the frequency and severity of pain-triggered chain reactions.

By practicing pain and stress management interventions, you may be able to prevent pain-triggered reactions from occurring altogether.

It is entirely possible to experience and witness pain, and still have a rich, full, and meaningful life.

Answer this question: Are you *living* with pain, or are you *suffering* from pain? You can choose to accept and cradle pain. You can gently lean into it. And by shifting your perceptions, you can let go of suffering.

Perceptions matter. Yes, there are horrific diseases. Yes, patients can be rude. And yes, some supervisors are more easy-going than others. But most of the time, it isn't the work you do that's stressful – it's your *perception* of the work you do. Most of the time, the people you interact with aren't threatening – it's your *perception* of those people that makes them a threat. In fact, perceptions are the actual cause of your muscle tension.

When someone claims his job is stressful or his boss is terrible, that person is unconsciously saying, *I'm a victim*. And compared to other misguided perceptions, victimhood is particularly disempowering. By definition, victims see themselves as blameless. They reject personal responsibility for their circumstances.

Burnout is the physical and mental exhaustion caused by long-term, emotionally demanding care giving. It's a product of the care you provide, and your workplace environment. Therefore, a broad range of factors can contribute to burnout, including charting demands, on-call duties, productivity expectations, performance reviews, Joint Commission surveys, and workplace culture.

Compassion fatigue is a numb, withdrawn emotional state that diminishes a caregiver's capacity to witness human suffering and to offer empathy.

What's the difference between compassion and empathy? Empathy is when you're aware of someone's feelings, followed by thoughts on how *you* might feel if confronting similar circumstances. Compassion, however, is when you have a clear understanding of someone's feelings; you accept those feelings; and you take action to help.

Cortisol is a steroid that builds up as a result of chronic stress. High levels of cortisol weaken the body's immune system and lead to muscle wasting. Cortisol increases blood sugar and causes fat to accumulate around the body's core. Vigorous, aerobic exercise is perhaps the best way to lower the body's cortisol level.

Studies show that chronic stress erodes and damages critical parts of human DNA. The longevity of each cell is compromised, thereby increasing the likelihood of a shorter lifespan.

★★★

You have two ways to breathe. One is the shallow breathing that comes from your chest, and the other is a deeper breathing that's supported by your diaphragm. Chest breathing stimulates the sympathetic nervous system. It puts your body and mind on high alert — as if there were an imminent threat to your safety. In contrast, diaphragm-supported breathing activates the parasympathetic nervous system which promotes calmness.

Are you breathing correctly? Here's a reminder of how to know for sure. Place your hand on your stomach as you breathe in and out. If you see and feel your hand move inward and outward with each breath, you know that your diaphragm is working the way you want it to. With practice, diaphragm-supported breathing will become your normal, natural, and preferred way to breathe.

★★★

Each day: Set aside 20 minutes for spiritual meditation, reflection, or prayer.

Each week: Take a silent, 60 minute walk in the woods. Or take several shorter walks that, when combined, total one hour. If you prefer, either yoga or tai chi is an excellent substitute.

Each week: If your health allows, do an aerobic activity such as jogging, rowing, swimming, bicycling, or power walking. Or choose to play a sport like basketball, racquetball, tennis, or soccer. Or participate in a group exercise led by an instructor. Aim for three, 30 to 40 minute workouts per week.

★★★

SCENARIO: In order to soothe your pain, you might indulge in over-eating, or you may drink excessively. These are obvious examples of harmful lifestyle choices. What's more, as poor choices become deeply imbedded, you're more likely to resist help.

INTERVENTION: In any environment, you have the power to be intentional, rather than reactional. You have the power to make healthy choices, rather than harmful ones. You can also reach out for help by contacting a professional counselor. Or, you can seek advice from a colleague at work, someone you trust and admire. Additionally, you can develop and follow a detailed self-care plan.

★★★

SCENARIO: Care giving can bring constant interruptions to the time you spend *away* from work, the time you spend at home with family. There's always one more email to answer, or one more work-related phone call to make.

INTERVENTION: Establish reasonable boundaries and strive to keep them. When you enjoy your time at home and get the rest you need, you'll be a better caregiver the following day.

★★★

SCENARIO: You're feeling frustrated. You haven't been given the resources needed to handle the demands of your job.

INTERVENTION: Think of it this way. There's only one thing a supervisor can *demand* of you: to do your best. By choosing to do your best, you are honoring your patients, your employer, yourself, and your Covenant. Finally, ask this question: *How can I possibly feel frustrated when I'm doing my best?*

★★★

SCENARIO: You are so anxious and stressed right now, you're not sure you will be able to make that last patient visit this afternoon.

INTERVENTION: When feeling stressed, anxious, and tense, close your eyes and let go of all thoughts. Focus your mind on breathing in and out. Slowly inhale while silently counting to five. Then slowly exhale as you silently count to five. Breathe deeply using your diaphragm. Relax your pelvic floor muscles. Repeat this three times.

Next, do a body scan, from head to toe. Identify tense muscles and allow them to soften. Relax any muscles that are squeezed or clenched. Continue to take deep, cleansing breaths until your anxiety subsides.

Try asking God for calmness: *Gracious God, help me feel your presence and peace.*

Or, try shifting your self-talk ...

- "I've experienced these feelings before, and I've always been able to persevere. I will persevere again."
- "I am strong, confident, and adaptable."
- "I choose to dismiss all doubt and negativity."
- "I embrace the reality that I am safe and I am loved."

After you're relaxed and refocused, you'll be more compassionate and effective for that last patient visit of the day.

★★★

SCENARIO: You awaken in the morning and don't know if you're able to go to work. You don't know if you have anything left to give.

INTERVENTION: When having negative thoughts and doubts about your work, revisit your Covenant. Then, reflect on the positive aspects of your job, such as ...

"It's an honor to serve the sick and the dying."

"My career glorifies God."

"I'm making a real difference in people's lives."

"Yes, I work hard – but I'm grateful for my job and all that it provides, including a salary and benefits."

★★★

SCENARIO: You feel tension in your back, shoulder, and neck muscles.

INTERVENTION: Relax your body's muscles through self-regulation. First, complete a total body scan. Next, identify tense muscles. Then, relax and soften them. With practice, this three-step intervention will take about 60 seconds. Try doing it once or twice an hour. Remember, no squeezing or clenching!

★★★

QUESTION: Do you have what it takes to be a hospice caregiver for the next twenty years?

ANSWER: Only time will tell. But if you hope to have a long and rewarding hospice career, consider the following advice ...

- Adjust your perceptions of pain, suffering, death, and dying.
- See the world as neutral and your environment as safe.
- Make sure your work is Covenant-driven.
- Rely on self-approval, rather than approval from others.
- Let go of making judgments.
- Understand that you can't control every outcome.
- Don't take things personally.
- Strike a balance between confidence and humility.
- Be honest about your weaknesses.
- Be tolerant of growing pains.
- Develop a strong peer support network.
- Practice self-care diligently.

★★★

In a support group of peers, it is safe to …

Talk about your trauma.

Share your thoughts and feelings about your work.

Disclose your weaknesses.

Accept support.

Receive guidance.

★★★

Your bedside care is a ministry that's touching hearts and lives in a positive way. You build trust-based relationships with your patients by creating a safe, sacred space at the bedside. Your work is making the world a better place – it's making a positive difference in more ways than you know.

★★★

Hospice caregivers have a servant's heart. Is there a greater gift, a better blessing?

★★★

Kindness and compassion are the human manifestations of God's mercy and grace.

★★★

Your mind will see threats and dangers where there are none. Moreover, your mind will urge you to examine the worst case scenario for every set of circumstances. And while these perils are merely illusions, they act as stressors nonetheless. Mark Twain wrote, "I've lived through a thousand catastrophes, and three of them actually happened."

★★★

When you become aware of a negative thought, try this three-step process. And if you find it helpful, add this technique to your coping toolbox.

1. First, realize that you're fixated on a negative thought, a past regret, or a future worry.
2. Next, release that thought, regret, or worry just like you would drop a "hot potato."
3. Then, quickly focus your attention on a sensory experience, something in your immediate field of awareness that you can actually see, touch, hear, taste, or smell. This third step keeps the unwanted thought from returning.

★★★

Therapists have long recognized the effectiveness of an anxiety relieving technique called Paradoxical Intention. This method relies on humor to ease tension. Here's how it works ...

A public speaker might face his audience and begin by saying, "During my last speech, I became light-headed. This time, I intend to pass out."

A nurse who's preparing to draw blood could say to the patient, "I did this for the first time yesterday. But don't worry, I have experience now."

A chaplain who's been asked to offer a prayer might start by saying, "My last prayer only lasted thirty minutes. I hope to go for an hour this time."

★★★

WATCH YOUR HABITS AND IMPROVE YOUR HEALTH

Eating healthy foods doesn't mean you're on a special diet; it's just a sensible choice to make.

Your body will tell you if you're eating too much of certain foods and not enough of others. So it pays to listen closely to what your body is saying.

If you're consuming too much caffeine, possible side effects include jitters, an elevated heartbeat, and a hard time falling asleep. Additionally, you might experience heartburn or stomach pains.

Too much salt can result in fluid retention. Moreover, research indicates that a high sodium diet may lead to increased confusion or overall cognitive decline.

If you're eating too many saturated fats, possible side effects include constipation, acid reflux, heartburn, and increased forgetfulness.

Consuming too much sugar can lead to mood swings, fatigue, high blood pressure, and blood sugar spikes.

Lean meat provides the protein your body needs. If you choose to follow a vegetarian diet, make sure you're getting enough Vitamin B12. Eggs and fortified tofu are great choices.

If you're always hungry or chronically tired, you may want to eat more "good" fats. Olive oil is a healthy food that may work well for you. Evidence suggests that good fats boost learning and memory skills too.

Salmon is heralded as an excellent source of omega-3 fatty acids, which are good for your heart. And salmon is also rich in Vitamin D, known for boosting your body's immune system and bone strength. If you can't quite recover from a cold – or if you have achy bones, muscles, or joints – then you may have a Vitamin D shortage. Along with fish, you could try adding low fat milk to your diet.

Vitamin C is another immune system enhancer. Citrus fruits and juices are a natural source of Vitamin C, an absolute must for maintaining your body's health. In addition, citrus fruits and leafy green veggies are rich with folic acid, the B vitamin needed to produce serotonin – a critical neurotransmitter and mood stabilizer.

Finally, low fiber diets are linked to a number of uncomfortable maladies, including constipation, bloating, and bowel irritation. Eating enough high-fiber foods – like lentils, for instance – can help you avoid these nagging problems.

Bonus tips ...

Almonds are a great choice for boosting your energy and strengthening your immune system.

Fresh fruits and vegetables provide the antioxidants your body uses to combat disease and premature aging.

The superfood category is a menu of nature's healthiest edibles. The following list includes some of the superfoods you expect to see, as well as a few tasty and beneficial treats that may surprise you: garlic, peppermint, ginger, black pepper, walnuts, beets, tomatoes, onions, spinach, broccoli, kale, blueberries, black raspberries, guava, and papaya.

★★★

If you're looking to lose a few pounds, cutting back on carbohydrates might be an attractive option. Your body turns carbs, primarily starches and sugars, into fat. So if you're willing to eat fewer pasta and potato dishes, and go easy on the breads and sweets, those extra pounds will start melting away. You can eat enough fish, poultry, eggs, nuts, cheese, and salads – with low-carb dressing – to not feel hungry. Eggs and cheese provide essential fatty acids. Other healthy proteins include beans, soy, and low-fat dairy products.

Try eating strawberries, raspberries, and blueberries topped with a small dollop of whipped cream rather than more traditional, sugar-laden desserts. A low-carb diet "tricks" your body into burning its reserves instead of any newly consumed calories. The clinical term is ketosis, a normal metabolic process whereby fat is burned whenever your body doesn't have sufficient carbohydrate intake. As an added bonus, consuming less sugar promotes healthy A1C blood levels, thus lowering your risk of becoming diabetic. As for carbs, you can't go wrong with eating fruits, vegetables, and high-fiber whole grains.

Still, there's a downside. Following a strict, low-carb diet for longer than a few months could stress your body, or possibly lead to painful kidney stones. A more prudent, long-term approach is to monitor and limit your overall carb intake. This can be achieved by estimating the carbs you consume. For most women, a desirable target is around forty-five carbs per meal. Men usually do well by limiting their carbs to about sixty per meal. In addition to your three main meals, you can eat two, fifteen carb snacks. That way, you'll avoid frequent blood sugar spikes. These are sustainable goals which typically enhance overall health and vitality.

For most healthy men and women, a high-protein diet isn't harmful, especially when it's just for a short time. However a long-term, high-protein diet could cause headaches or constipation, and could also increase the risk of heart or kidney disease. Talk to your doctor before you start a new diet, adopt a new exercise routine, or make a major lifestyle change.

★★★

If you're open to an "outside-the-box" method to curb your appetite or to lose weight, then start by reading the following ground rules.

1. Understand that, within a tolerable period of time, hunger pangs subside whether you choose to eat or not.
2. You can change your mind and alter your perception of any hunger sensations you may experience, and meditation is one of the best techniques available to help you turn negative associations into positive ones.
3. Realize that it's your choice to eat or not to eat. Moreover, you control the kinds of food you consume and the portions as well.

Next, try this ...

Abstain from eating until you're feeling hungry and are experiencing sensations like a "growling" stomach. Then, close your eyes and focus on the physical sensations of hunger. But instead of perceiving these sensations as undesirable, do the exact opposite: welcome, embrace, cherish, and celebrate them! While meditating, tell yourself that you want *more* of these hunger feelings and *more* of these hunger experiences. Convince yourself – your mind – that you just can't get enough of these sensations and experiences, knowing all the while that they will gradually fade away. Remind yourself of the power and control you have in choosing when, what, and how much you eat. Try to maintain an intensely focused meditation for at least fifteen minutes. Then repeat this process once a day for seven consecutive days. After that, do a "reinforcement" meditation once a week.

Keep in mind that your goal is not to be fasting for days on end, or to stop eating altogether. The objective is to reduce your intake of calories by choosing to eat modest portions of healthy foods – and to integrate this lifestyle change without thinking that you're suffering or making a big sacrifice.

For additional motivation, paste a picture of your face onto a picture of someone's body that you find attractive. Then, put this "new you" photo in a place where it's easy to access. Each morning, look at it for a minute or so. Visualizing the weight loss that you're striving to achieve will remind you of your long-term goal, and help manifest this transformation.

Bonus tip: Before eating a meal, remember to offer a blessing. A blessing not only expresses gratitude, it can prevent an unpleasant experience, like nausea.

★★★

Are you looking to achieve or maintain a target weight? Keep a food diary! Studies show that writing down what you eat may reveal patterns and insights you're unaware of. This added information might put you on the path to improved health. Whether you use a notebook, a computer, or a smart phone, write down everything you eat and drink – and do it after each meal or snack. Then, review your eating and drinking habits at the end of the day. Even if that's all you do, it will help you be a more mindful eater. For instance, you might find yourself thinking: *Wow, I ate 14 chocolate chip cookies today. I had no idea. Or, Hmm … I finished three 20 ounce bottles of Pepsi today. I'm surprised I drank that much.* Here's the key. Don't feel guilty or beat yourself up about it. Just be *aware* of what you're actually eating and drinking. The awareness alone will prompt you to make healthier choices.

If you're willing to take this method to the next level, you can:

- Write down *when* you eat and drink. This will provide additional knowledge. Do you tend to skip a certain meal? Try replacing it with a mini-meal or snack. Does your appetite roar as bedtime approaches? Perhaps a modest but yummy treat will tame that growling stomach.

- Make a note describing your *activities* during mealtimes. Do you forget to eat when you're focused on work? Then, set an alarm to remind you. Are you on your phone or watching TV while you eat? It's easy to consume too much when you're distracted, so try creating a distraction free zone while eating your meals.
- Finally, record how you are *feeling* when you eat. Are you consuming food and beverages as a way to cope with stress, sadness, or boredom? If so, then address what's bothering you more directly. For example, choose to exercise when you're feeling stressed. Reach out to a friend if you're feeling sad. Or pursue a fun hobby when you're feeling bored.

★★★

Closing reflection …

Write down three ways that your work as a caregiver has improved your life. Next, write down three ways that your care giving work has negatively affected your life. How would your life be changed if you could diminish, or possibly eliminate, the negative aspects of your work? From your list, choose one negative issue – the negative that you're most interested in eliminating. Reflect on it. What can you do differently to diminish or eliminate this negative? How can you implement this change right now?

★★★

DAY EIGHTEEN

GOD WINKS

> Everything in this life has purpose. There are no
> mistakes or coincidences; all events are blessings
> given to us to learn from. *Elisabeth Kubler-Ross*

★★★

God-wink events, situations, or circumstances defy randomness and
statistical probability. Moreover, they touch our hearts in a meaningful
way. A God-wink moment is a reminder that ours is an interconnected
world – that billions of life journeys are unfolding and intersecting
under the watchful eye of a Higher Power.

★★★

Born in South Korea and abandoned by their family, sisters Meagan and
Holly ended up at different orphanages. Their separation occurred when
the girls were too young to have memories of one another. Eventually,
each little girl was raised in America by different parents. At age forty-
five, Meagan landed a job at a hospital in Sarasota, Florida. There, she
was introduced to Holly, a coworker who was also South Korean. The
two women quickly noticed some intriguing parallels in their lives. Both
were licensed nursing assistants. There was just a one-year age difference;
and each of them had been adopted by an American family.

Finally, Meagan asked, "What was your last name when you were born?"
Holly replied, "Shin." As Meagan's eyes grew wide, she exclaimed, "That
was my last name too!" By now, their similarities appeared to be more
than just coincidence, and the results of a DNA test confirmed it: They
were sisters! After a 7,500 mile journey that took more than four decades,
Meagan and Holly were unexpectedly, but joyously, reunited. They met
working the same job, on the same shift, on the same floor, of the same

hospital. All of this happened without either of them knowing they had a sister. What are the odds?

★★★

Ellen was just seven years old when her mother, Josephine died. Memories were hazy, but Ellen knew that her mom, a writer and poet, once lived in New York City. Now, Ellen realized it was her turn to live in the Big Apple. Picking up a newspaper, she found an apartment for rent in Greenwich Village. A taxi dropped her off in front of an older, but attractive, brick building at 288 West 12th Street, and a kind gentleman escorted her to Apartment B and unlocked the door. Right away, Ellen felt drawn to the cozy living room that featured a fireplace. It was a welcoming space in which she could launch her own writing career. And the kitchen, though very small, had a window facing a lovely courtyard. She quickly told the landlord, "I'll take it!"

A week later, staring at a mountain of boxes, Ellen dreaded the chore of unpacking. But at the same time, it was a new beginning and her heart was filled with hope. In one of the boxes, she discovered the large envelope that held her mother's old papers and memorabilia. Ellen examined a few of the postcards and letters. Then, she found a poem which had her mom's name and address on it, a detail she hadn't noticed before: Josephine Blatt, 288-B West 12th Street, New York, New York. *Unbelievable,* she thought. *My mom lived in this same apartment!* Still holding that piece of paper, Ellen's hands began to tremble. As she recalls, "I was overcome by chills and tears. It couldn't be just a coincidence. I was comforted and was sure that I had landed in exactly the right place."

Adapted from a story by S. Rushnell

★★★

More than twenty years had passed since sisters and one-time best friends, Lois and Louise had spoken to one another. A bitter argument had left each of them hurting and unwilling to reconcile, even though they both lived in Sacramento. Listening to the radio, Lois heard about a Christmas Eve service sponsored by St. Paul's, a church she had never visited. Although it was a long drive, something compelled her to go. Lois, running a little late, arrived at the church and was surprised to find a large parking lot that was nearly full.

The usher who greeted Lois craned his neck to locate a pew that could hold one more guest. Finally, she was led to a spot where a long row of people scooted down and made enough space for her to be seated. After regaining her composure, Lois whispered to the woman next to her, "I'm glad I didn't get here any later." The woman turned her head and gasped, "Lois, is that you?" Louise and Lois had, in a most unlikely set of circumstances, been reunited. Following the service, the astonished sisters held hands and laughed. Louise explained that she, too, was visiting St. Paul's for the first time. Neither of them could remember what they had argued about so long ago, but the sisters were happy just to be friends again.

★★★

By design, the universe is like a giant, reflective sphere: We receive what we give. We harvest what we plant. Sometimes, this reality plays out figuratively. Other times, it's more literal – as found in the following true story …

Physician Michael Shannon was driving on a familiar highway, a route he took to Dana Point Harbor every Tuesday morning. Once there, he always joined a friend and, together, they walked a trail that followed the contours of the Pacific Ocean. But this Tuesday morning was unlike the previous ones. Without warning, a large truck pulled onto the road in front of Michael. There was no time to react. He recalls it this way: "I remember a sudden impact and the sound of breaking glass. Then, everything was still, like the whole world had stopped." Michael smelled smoke, and his feet and legs felt hot; but he was trapped in the wreckage, unable to move.

By chance, a team from the Orange County Fire Department, including paramedic Chris Trokey, was nearby. They arrived on the scene within two minutes. Chris, an eight-year veteran, quickly recognized the seriousness of the situation. The entire front end of the car was wedged beneath the semi's trailer. Even more alarming, flames were shooting from the car's engine. The rescue squad extinguished the fire and called for backup – stronger tools were needed to free the car's driver. Chris was struck by how this man had stayed remarkably calm: "He wasn't freaked out or screaming. He simply asked us to help him get out of the car. He said his name was Michael Shannon."

The second crew arrived and used the Jaws-of-Life to pry open the car door. Michael was strapped to a gurney and rushed to Mission Hospital, where Chris had asked the medical trauma team to be ready. He stayed with Michael in the back of the ambulance; and during their trip to the hospital, Chris silently thought, *Michael Shannon, that name is so familiar. Have I met this man before? Is he the same man who saved my life thirty years ago?*

Chris was a preemie who was born in the very same hospital they were headed to. Weighing only three pounds, two ounces, doctors told Chris's parents that their son had a 50-50 chance of surviving. But there was one devoted physician who wouldn't give up, a pediatrician named Michael Shannon. On some nights, he chose to sleep at the hospital by Chris's side. Perhaps the doctor's presence offered comfort during that fragile time, comfort which a struggling baby would feel, but not remember. Now, at thirty years old and six feet tall, Chris looked nothing like his first few weeks of life. So it wasn't surprising that Michael hadn't recognized him.

It took several weeks for Michael to recover, and Chris visited him daily. Both men were amazed as they talked about such an unlikely string of events. Michael helped Chris at a critical moment in his life; then Chris returned the favor by helping Michael at an equally critical time. Though neither man was particularly religious, their unexpected reconnection left them trusting in a Higher Power.

Adapted from a story by Lisa Miller

★★★

Another true story ...

There was nothing unusual about that winter's day in rural Wisconsin. Tammy was driving on a country road with her three Labradors – Lily, Molly, and Luke – nestled in the backseat. Tammy didn't see the patch of ice that caused her SUV to spin out of control. A moment later, she was thrown from her vehicle. A neighbor found Tammy – unconscious and critically injured – lying in the snow. Here's what happened.

The dogs were not hurt; and after the crash, they quickly escaped from the SUV. Molly stayed at Tammy's side, while Lily and Luke ran down the road. They discovered a house about one-half mile from the accident. Both dogs barked and scratched at the front door. As the homeowner emerged, Luke grabbed the man's sleeve and pulled him closer to the road. From this vantage point, he could see the overturned vehicle. The neighbor rushed to the scene and found Tammy lying motionless in the snow. He used his cell phone to call 911. Paramedics arrived and transported her to the closest hospital. Fortunately, Tammy recovered from her injuries.

There are, of course, different ways to view this sequence of events. One scenario, which is perfectly reasonable for many people, goes something like this. The dogs realize that Tammy is hurt and needs assistance. They love her and, knowing they can't save Tammy by themselves, one dog stands guard while the other two run down the road in search of someone who can help. Approaching a nearby house, the dogs consciously bark and scratch at the front door in order to alert anyone who might be inside. When a man opens the door, Luke understands that he must guide this person to a spot where the accident can be seen.

Others, however, may perceive things differently. They might believe the dog that stayed with Tammy was just resting and recovering from its trauma. The two dogs that ran down the road may have done so simply because they were terrified and wanted to put some distance between themselves and the accident site. Perhaps their barking and scratching at the neighbor's front door didn't have a strategic purpose. Rather, the dogs had unconsciously learned to bark and scratch at structures in which humans are likely to be found. And perhaps Luke often greets people by grabbing a sleeve and playing tug-of-war. After all, Labradors are known for being playful and putting things in their mouths.

Both views are merely different interpretations of the same story. To be honest, we don't know what dogs are actually thinking. Although it's unlikely that dogs analyze situations exactly as humans do, most dog owners are deeply grateful for one thing: the unconditional love they receive from their devoted canine companions. A final note: Tammy's drama was so compelling, the Wisconsin Veterinary Medical Association inducted her Labradors into its Hero Hall of Fame. These doctors were confident that Lily, Molly, and Luke understood, on some level, that Tammy was badly injured and needed help.

Veterinarians know that dogs are highly social animals – one of the few species where individuals will sacrifice their lives in order to save a member of the pack. Moreover, dogs have evolved to be creative problem solvers and nurturing team players. In other words, just because an altruistic interpretation of a story triggers warm and fuzzy feelings, doesn't mean the conclusion isn't accurate.

Adapted from *For the Love of a Dog* by Patricia McConnell

★★★

Closing Reflection ...

Some people see proof of God's love just about everywhere they look. Yet, as *A Course in Miracles* points out, "No amount of evidence can convince you of the truth you do not want." What do you choose to see? Do you notice the good, or the bad; the beautiful, or the ugly? When looking at the world, do you see evidence of a Higher Power? Reflect on how you've reached your conclusion. Have you ever felt a

Divine presence at the bedside of a patient? If so, try to describe that feeling.

★★★

DAY NINETEEN

DAVID R. HAWKINS

> Rare is the man who discovers truth; and the man
> who recognizes it is rarer still. *Baruch Spinoza*

★★★

By nearly any measure, David R. Hawkins, MD, PhD stands among the most accomplished men of his generation. He was an internationally renowned psychiatrist, researcher, author, humanitarian, and master teacher. Born in Milwaukee on June 3, 1927, Hawkins graduated from the Medical College of Wisconsin. He then moved to the East Coast, where his private practice quickly became the largest mental health clinic in New York City. Hawkins offered care to the city's most vulnerable men and women: individuals who were struggling with psychoses, addictions, homelessness, and abusive relationships. Later, he recalled, "Many of my patients were unfamiliar with respect and dignity, and some had never experienced love. I was their last hope, and no one was turned away."

Hawkins lectured at prominent universities and medical schools around the world, and he co-wrote a treatise on brain chemistry with Nobel laureate, Linus Pauling. His groundbreaking book on human consciousness, *Power vs. Force*, has been translated into twenty-five languages. A profound trust in God was foundational to his life and work. Hawkins chose to spend his last years in Sedona, Arizona – a location known for its remarkable beauty and tranquility.

★★★

Dr. Hawkins understood that two things account for much of the suffering associated with the human condition, both past and present. First, consciousness drives human behavior, shaping our thoughts, perceptions, words, and actions. This explains why humanity has always been plagued by war, crime, poverty, corruption, greed, ignorance, and so on. Secondly, when truth and falsehood are presented with equal conviction, the human mind cannot distinguish one from the other. This clarifies why history keeps repeating itself.

Through his research, Hawkins discovered that, collectively, the human experience unfolds in an algorithmic consciousness range of 100 to 600. More to the point, he learned that individuals who are functioning at a low level of consciousness – 200 or less – are perceiving life through a lens of fear, anger, misery, and hopelessness. They are consumed by guilt and shame. And for such people, God is a deity of punishment, vengeance, and condemnation. Unfortunately, a significant percentage of the world's population falls into this range.

On a more positive note, a large segment of humanity is functioning in the 200 to 400 range of consciousness, and these people hold a life-view shaped by meaning, purpose, and hope. They are justifiably proud of their achievements. Moreover, their God is merciful and inspiring.

Finally, there's a relatively small percentage of individuals around the world who are functioning in the 400 to 600 range of consciousness. These people see life as harmonious, whole, and perfect; and their God is benign, wise, and loving. They express gratitude for their gifts, and they are graced by inner peace.

This information allows us to make sense of the human condition. A basic understanding of consciousness not only helps us grasp why global problems are ongoing, we gain new insights as to why our world is blessed by kindness, compassion, and love. Hawkins determined that both individual and collective levels of human consciousness are gradually – but steadily – growing in the right direction. This offers genuine hope for our future.

★★★

Hawkins also discovered that individual life forms are born with a potentiality, and then evolve spontaneously to a level of actualization. What's more, each one-of-a-kind journey unfolds in an environment of Divine Order. Hawkins believed that this principle holds true for humans, too. In our case, intentionality drives us to attain an elevated level of consciousness.

★★★

God is timeless and changeless. Yet, one's perception of God is ever-evolving.

★★★

Transformative opportunities arise from time to time in one's life. Usually, these seminal moments occur during a time of crisis, or a season of hardship.

★★★

What seems erudite to one level of consciousness might be seen as naive or even destructive when viewed through the lens of a higher level of consciousness.

★★★

A higher level of consciousness doesn't make one person better, or superior, to another. What it does mean, however, is that the more conscious person has a better concept of reality. Accordingly, this more grounded person offers a better example of how God wishes us to live; for such a person is more receptive to spirit guidance and empowerment. An individual's behavior is the most reliable indicator of consciousness.

A genuinely kind and loving person is, by definition, functioning at a high level of consciousness.

***

There's a paradox within heightened consciousness. As humans collectively achieve higher levels of enlightenment, God seems to be, at times, more distant than ever. Our developing minds produce a relentless stream of obstructive thoughts, and God's very existence is doubted. Yet, once humanity emerges from its valley of disillusionment – after vanquishing our sense of separation and calming our busy minds – we can grow exponentially closer to our Creator. Collectively, we will have the potential to connect with God in a way that was never before possible.

***

Striking similarities abound in the animal kingdom. For instance, horses and zebras clearly share many outward appearances. Yet, while resembling one another, these close relatives are two distinct species. That's why you won't find a striped horse or a dappled zebra. So the burning question is: How are new species formed on our planet?

It's true that sudden and random mutations are part of organic life, as are gradual and purposeful adaptations. But do such phenomena explain how countless species – and their incredible diversity – have come to populate the world? Naturalists suggest that, in fact, undiscovered species far outnumber those we've identified to date. And as additional flora and fauna are cataloged, we often can't tell if a new discovery has existed for ages, or just for a short while. Is it a life form that's thriving, or on the brink of extinction?

In studies related to his consciousness research, Hawkins gained surprising insights on the origin of new species – a perplexing mystery that has intrigued scientists for centuries. His conclusion: New plant and animal species appear spontaneously within our natural environment of Divine grace. Think of it this way. At the perfect moment and at the optimal place, a new branch appears on the tree of life. Simply stated, life on earth is the result of God's love and Divine Order. And upon further reflection, how could it be otherwise?

★★★

David R. Hawkins: Thoughts and reflections ...

In an effort to understand the incomprehensible, people typically rely on linear thinking, such as: *If I witness a miracle, then I will believe there's a God.* Yet, life itself is nonlinear; and as a result, humanity is stuck in a cycle of intellectual frustration.

You change the world not by what you say or do, but as a consequence of what you become.

To become more conscious is the greatest gift a person can give. Moreover, in a ripple effect, the gift comes back to its source.

Spiritual growth is not an accomplishment, but a way of life.

Through all-inclusive, unconditional compassion, the world is healed.

When it comes to solving social problems, support a solution instead of attacking the presumed cause.

We exist and survive, not because of the ego, but in spite of it.

What the ego cannot lift with all its might is like a feather to the grace of God.

By design, the pathway to God is not easy. The journey requires considerable courage, fortitude, and willingness – strengthened by humility.

Holding a goal in mind is helpful, because what is held in mind tends to actualize. Potentiality manifests as actuality through intention and commitment.

Stubbornness is defined by the man who insists his Venus flytrap can become a vegetarian.

The ego relishes opportunities to rewrite history. By judging content and ignoring context, heroes are vilified and bravery is condemned.

It isn't necessary to drive yourself forward. Advance as roadblocks are removed. Thus, you are attracted by the future rather than propelled by the past.

The love of God shines equally on all.

As each worry arises, surrender it to God.

What you see reflects your thinking; and your thinking reflects your choice of what you see.

You are powerless without God's help. Yet, the moment you call upon Divinity, you summon forth that power.

Love is a state of awareness, a way of seeing and treating others and oneself.

Humility amounts to dropping pride and pretense, and accepting that fallibility is a normal human characteristic.

The readiness to initiate a journey to God cannot be forced, nor should people be faulted if the idea has not occurred to them as yet. Their level of consciousness must advance to the point where such a journey is meaningful and attractive.

New creations are born of Divine grace. Moreover, such spontaneous births are new species, not hybrids or mutations. New species have arrived this way over and over again since the beginning of time.

There is nothing like the joy of experiencing God's loving presence.

★★★

Closing reflection ...

Empowered by choice, I will strive to be more easygoing, forgiving, kind, and loving towards life in all of its expressions, including myself. I will try to be helpful and to respect everyone I meet, without exception. I trust the love, mercy, and wisdom of God – who understands that I have limitations and that I make mistakes. I place my faith in a forgiving Creator whose grace has no boundaries. Through passionate discipline, I will transcend negativity by making positive choices. With God's help, I will relinquish demoralizing thoughts, and I will abolish destructive behaviors.

★★★

First, the ego will invent a problem. Next, the ego will brag about its clever solution. Yet, neither the problem nor the solution is real. Look closely at your current worries. Are they real, or not? Dismiss the self-created conflicts. And for the remaining ones, give patience and trust an opportunity to solve them.

★★★

Faith isn't just a concept or an idea; it is something you should *live*. Your faith should be expressed by every thought, word, and deed.

★★★

DAY TWENTY

BOUNDARIES

Good fences make good neighbors. *Robert Frost*

★★★

Borders and boundaries are an integral part of the human experience: a wall, roof, door, or fence; a wallet or purse; a private phone number or a computer password. Cities, counties, states, and nations maintain borders. You keep a personal space between yourself and others, even among your closest friends. Cultural customs and courtesies are honored in public places. Ethics and morals offer guidelines for appropriate behavior. Laws and law enforcement are designed to establish order. Without such borders, life would be chaotic. Indeed, anarchy would replace civility.

★★★

Nature, too, has boundaries: mountains, canyons, and deserts; rivers, lakes, and oceans.

★★★

A church, a synagogue, a mosque, a temple, an ashram – each one is a boundary, a haven for worshipers.

★★★

Caregivers must have boundaries as well. Otherwise, burnout is inevitable.

★★★

A boundary is simply a limit, or a clear space. Ideally, caregivers should establish boundaries that promote balance and space between life at work, and life at home. Additionally, boundaries should promote a clearly defined space between caregivers and their patients. While helpful limits are often psychological in nature, physical boundaries – such as rules against inappropriate touching – are equally important. Boundaries like these express respect and professionalism. And this might surprise you: Research indicates that caregivers who maintain a reasonable work–life balance are the happiest *and* the most productive. Therefore, limits and boundaries are good for both staff *and* employers!

★★★

It's a myth that you must sacrifice superior job performance in order to take care of yourself. In fact, the opposite is true. You must take care of yourself in order to excel at work. With that in mind, wellness coach, Abby Quillen recommends the following guidelines for setting boundaries at work ...

Clarify what you value. Do some soul-searching. What is really important to you? What are your highest needs? What do you deserve in life? Your answers can be used to guide and shape the boundaries you choose to adopt.

Create rules and structure. Try to stop work at the same time each day. Step away from your work area during breaks. Limit your accessibility on days off. Avoid workplace romance. And no gossiping.

Write down your boundaries. The process of using pen and paper to write down your boundaries will help you remember them better. Rules that are more entrenched in your mind are more likely to be followed.

Track your time. Although laptops, tablets, and smart phones are time savers, they also blur the line between work and home. Is work creeping into your personal life? Are excessive demands straining your relationships or keeping you from pursuing other interests? If so, consider limiting after-hours work, and set aside one day per week to completely unplug.

Communicate clearly and directly. On occasions when you need to explain your boundaries to others, be clear, direct, calm, confident, and respectful. Also, try to present your rules and limits in a positive manner. It isn't always easy; but the more you work at improving your communication skills, the better you will get. In other words, practice saying, *No.* And after your boundaries are understood by the people around you, remember that actions speak louder than words. If you ever feel overwhelmed, schedule a meeting with your supervisor to revisit your tasks and priorities. Do you need to improve your time management skills? Is there a teammate who can step in temporarily to ease your workload?

Expect violations and compromises. An ideal boundary is firm but not rigid. Once you set a healthy limit, be as consistent as possible at keeping that promise to yourself. But if you need to compromise occasionally, don't feel bad. A little flexibility is okay.

★★★

It's important to have a meaningful connection between caregiver and patient. To achieve this goal, offer your patients unconditional regard and respect. That said, you must maintain a proper boundary between self and patient.

★★★

Caregivers typically react to fear, shock, and horror in one of three ways: moral outrage, disassociation, or numbness. Coincidentally, these reactions are identical to the fear responses of wild animals: fight, flight, or freeze.

★★★

Caregiver boundary tips ...

1. Stay grounded in the present moment.
2. Be aware of your intention and goal.
3. Center yourself first; then serve your patient.

4. Remain aware of your role.
5. Engage the patient at the beginning.
6. Close your visit at the end.

★★★

Beware of falling into the trap of counter-transference — when a caregiver projects personal feelings onto a patient. For instance, a female nurse could be visiting a male patient whose appearance or mannerisms remind the nurse of her own father. Without an awareness of this association — and the discipline required to maintain a professional boundary — the nurse may develop feelings for her patient that mirror the feelings she has for her father.

Transference, on the other hand, is a potential hazard for patients. To offer an example of transference, let's use the flip side of the first scenario. In other words, transference might unfold like this: A female nurse visits a male patient. The patient notices that the nurse reminds him of his own daughter. Soon, the patient develops emotional ties to the nurse — projected feelings that are similar to the ones he has for his daughter.

Here's the takeaway. Monitor your feelings and emotions. You might ask, *Are my feelings for Mr. Smith appropriate? Am I keeping an adequate boundary?* And while you can't control the feelings that your patients experience, you can lessen the risk of misguided attachments by simply redirecting patient conversations to clinical issues. Also, remember to place strict limits on the personal information you share. Here's the good news. You can implement these reasonable safeguards and continue to have friendly, cheerful, and rewarding patient interactions.

★★★

What could possibly go wrong when a caregiver ignores professional boundaries? Consider that hypothetical scenario where a female nurse is visiting a male patient who resembles her own father. If the nurse had offered this patient personal information about her family and her real father during the first visit, then a similar conversation would likely occur during her next visit with this patient. Very quickly, the nurse could develop a strong emotional attachment. Then, how would the nurse respond to his decline? Would she react as if her real father were declining? And what feelings might the nurse experience if this patient were to die? Would she grieve as if he were an actual family member? Finally, what if a nurse routinely becomes attached to her patients in such a way? How might that impact a long-term hospice career?

★★★

As a hospice caregiver, one of your goals is to manage each patient's pain. Yet, some patients refuse to take pain medicine, and suffer because of it. That choice is an example of self-determined end-of-life care. It's a choice that every patient of sound mind has the right to make. When patients choose to suffer, realize that it's *their* journey and *their* choice. If it were your journey, *you* would be the patient – and have the right to make a different choice.

★★★

Remember that you're a caregiver, not a judge. Your suffering begins the moment you label an event as unfortunate or undesirable. What might happen if you were to resist the temptation of judging life's circumstances?

★★★

Closing reflection ...

Why is it important for caregivers to establish clear boundaries? The answer is simple. Reasonable rules keep your personal life from interfering with your work, and prevent your work from intruding on your personal life. In truth, realistic boundaries help you achieve work-life excellence.

Take a moment to write down three boundaries that you would like to keep at work. Reflect on how you will benefit by honoring these boundaries. In your mind, create a hypothetical scenario for each boundary – a work situation where you tactfully maintain your "limit" or "clear space." This exercise will help you successfully resolve a real boundary problem when it arises.

★★★

Here's an idea. If you have a dedicated cell phone for work, make a point to turn it off and put it in a drawer when you get home – presuming that you're not on call. And do the same for a job-related tablet or laptop computer. By literally placing these and similar items out of sight, your thoughts are less likely to be centered on work issues.

Try to think of another practical innovation that will clarify your boundaries and promote work-life excellence.

★★★

DAY TWENTY-ONE

THE HUMAN CONDITION

> If you can adopt a mindset which accepts worldwide
> human suffering, it will help counteract your feelings
> of unhappiness and discontent. *Dalai Lama*

★★★

Why does a book on wellness and harmony include an examination of sociological, ideological, and apocalyptic themes? As it happens, a person's perception of the human condition will shape his or her worldview, which raises a key question: Is your worldview influenced by optimism, or pessimism? The answer is important because your perspective of the world – be it positive or negative – will inevitably sway your demeanor both at home and at work.

An optimistic worldview promotes an underlying sense that all is well. But even if you tend to be a pessimist, there's encouraging news. Perceptions are nothing more than choices. So if you have a negative worldview, you can choose to see the human condition differently. You can, for example, focus on positive things, such as convincing statistical evidence that points to less poverty and fewer wars in today's world. So now, through a lens of historical and sociological context, let's take a thoughtful look at humanity and our planet.

★★★

Humans spend a great deal of time judging things. We judge people and events. We pronounce judgments on the past and the present. Nonetheless, we remain inept. In truth, we've barely achieved a beginner's level of judicial competence. This deficiency stems, in part, from focusing heavily on content, while largely ignoring context. To better understand this phenomenon, let's look closer at our checkered past.

Early humans were tribal by nature and, more often than not, the tribes were at war with one another. Each tribe focused on defeating its perceived adversaries. And always, the victors would annihilate the vanquished. Humanity carried on this way for thousands of years. Until one day, a victorious tribal leader had an intriguing idea: *Instead of killing my enemies, I will enslave them. They will build monuments that prove my greatness!*

The intention, of course, was reprehensible. Yet regardless of intentions, to *not* murder is a higher choice. To *not* murder is a choice that expresses mercy, even when the decision maker is unaware of it. Soon thereafter, enslaving defeated rivals – not killing them – became the norm. Today, the mere thought of slavery is repulsive. But during an early, brutal period of human evolution, perhaps enslaving people – rather than slaughtering them – was a misstep that ultimately served the greater good.

172

Next, let's look at a time when there were very few safety nets in human society. Think of the world as a Charles Dickens' novel. In other words, people who didn't have money were homeless and hungry. When someone borrowed money but couldn't repay it, he or she went to a debtor's prison. But things were starting to change. Great Britain's Industrial Revolution created a huge demand for workers. During that time, a selfish business owner had a compelling thought: *I can use children to produce my wares. I'll get them to work hard. Even better, I'll pay them next to nothing, thereby increasing my profit!*

Once again, the intent was despicable. But if you carefully examine the evolution of child labor in England, you'll discover a thread of mercy. For despite the meager wages, English children earned enough money to provide food for their elderly family members – those who were too weak or sick to work in a factory. If not for these working children, countless elders of that era would have starved to death. Could this be yet another misstep in human history that ultimately led to a better world?

★★★

God doesn't create painful experiences, but transforms them in a way that serves the greater good.

★★★

As a sidebar, the Industrial Revolution began in Great Britain and eventually became a global movement. Starting around 1760 and ending by 1840, the Industrial Revolution transformed humanity. Consumer goods were produced much more efficiently and, therefore, were more affordable. Cities grew, and jobs were plentiful. There were hundreds of new, labor-saving inventions; and historians agree that, for most people, day-to-day living was dramatically improved.

★★★

After communing with God, Moses knew that he couldn't lead his people to the Promised Land straightaway. The Israelites, after all, had been enslaved in Egypt for as long as they could remember. Moses understood that, if given too much freedom too quickly, his people would be tormented by anxiety. As slaves, the Israelites weren't familiar with making decisions; nor were they skilled at managing personal responsibilities – the accoutrements of liberty. Thus began a forty-year journey.

Their epic wandering provided enough time for a new generation to come of age, a generation of men and women who embraced freedom and opportunity. What's more, they didn't perceive themselves as victims of exploitation and abuse. Though they had listened to stories about slavery, this new generation had not *experienced* it. They were descendants of slaves, but they were *not* slaves. So when these young men and women finally entered the Promised Land, they were prepared for freedom and equipped to prosper.

★★★

Slavery, human trafficking, and child labor abuses continue to be global problems. However, more governments around the world are recognizing the inherent evil of these conditions and are taking steps to eradicate them. This bodes well for our future.

★★★

When judging the past, it's difficult to be fair – especially when context is overlooked.

★★★

Why do humans like to rewrite history? First, rewriting history is much easier than doing the work needed to gain accurate insights on previous eras. But more to the point, it's the only way to guarantee the desired outcome.

★★★

On some occasions, history is rewritten immediately. Other times, revisions may occur years, decades, or even centuries later.

★★★

Even as we stumble, humanity continues to take steps in the right direction. For by the grace of God, love always prevails.

★★★

Wherever you find people, you find problems. Note that poverty, crime, corruption, and war have been prominent throughout human history. And as long as people are driven by unabated anger and inflated egos; and as long as people are functioning at low levels of consciousness, pain and suffering will surely be linked to the human condition.

★★★

People functioning at low levels of consciousness rarely make positive contributions to humanity. Sometimes these individuals are benign, doing as little as possible. Other times, they are the perpetrators of violent crimes or acts of terror.

★★★

As you gain a greater understanding of the human condition, you acquire knowledge-based perspectives that empower you to cope more effectively with global suffering.

★★★

By adopting a more mature worldview, you begin to accept the certainty of human suffering. You start to let go of guilt, and realize that it's not your job to save humanity.

★★★

Freedom is empowering; it elevates the human condition and is in harmony with God's will.

★★★

When horrible things happen, remember that God did not create evil; nor is God the source of human pain and suffering. In truth, all creatures are born of God's love. Evil, then, is a product of human choices. An evil being is a soul at war with itself, with God, and with God's creations. Or think of it this way: Evil is a decision to deny the reality of love!

★★★

Passive resistance is an effective, nonviolent response to oppression and exploitation. Note that Mahatma Gandhi – a diminutive and gentle, but powerful man – brought the indomitable British Empire to its knees.

★★★

Historically, men have gained courage by engaging in hand-to-hand combat, while women have found courage by withstanding the rigors of childbirth.

★★★

War is the manifestation of conflicting ideologies.

★★★

In today's culture, news and social media have become the lens through which the world is perceived. And as false narratives are tirelessly promoted, more and more people are choosing to see themselves as victims. Yet, there *is* a remedy; for truth can defeat this perpetual cycle of grievances. And that's why spiritual teachers point out that the truth will set you free.

★★★

During the passage of time, certain nations and tribes have established and maintained peaceful relationships with their neighbors, while other nations and tribes have constantly been at war. Perhaps you've wondered, *Why do some groups of people get along, and others don't?*

For starters, peaceful nations and tribes might be benefiting from things such as lower population density, protective geographical barriers, or simply the good fortune of being surrounded by easy-going, like-minded humans. But if you dig deeper, you'll find that peaceful, freedom-based nations and tribes are led by men and women who have achieved higher levels of consciousness. These leaders look at the world and see abundance, rather than lack. They see opportunities instead of obstacles. They have learned how to thrive, not just survive. They love life, rather than fear it. And because they embrace inclusive ideologies, they strive to uplift and liberate their neighbors, not oppress and conquer them.

Still, there will always be nations and tribes led by those who are mired in hatred and jealousy, and consumed by power and greed. There will always be corrupt leaders who have not yet learned how to love or forgive. And because of this reality, there will always be areas of the world that are torn apart by war and violence.

★★★

Yes, God does favor some nations over others. Benevolent nations promote liberty, and their citizens enjoy the freedom God wishes them to have. Autocratic countries, however, are defying God's will by suppressing freedom and exploiting their citizens. So while oppressive countries may gain short-term victories, their governments are destined to crumble. Such nations ultimately collapse under the weight of injustice.

★★★

Perhaps you've heard that, in a decade or two, the earth will be uninhabitable. Here's what we know for sure. Since the birth of our planet, dramatic change has been a natural, evolutionary phenomenon. Think about all that's happened. Entire continents have split apart, and asteroids have gouged enormous craters in the earth's crust. There was a time when much of North America was underwater and, at one point, rainforests covered the South Pole.

We also know that just a single event, such as a large volcanic eruption, can alter the earth's environment for years. Thankfully, our planet is immensely resilient and, given enough time, it can recover from extraordinary trauma. And though humans can neither control nor manage the earth's evolutionary changes, people *can* adapt – and actually thrive – while confronting ominous circumstances.

★★★

For centuries, people have been confidently – but incorrectly – predicting the end of the world. Such forecasts are by no means a new phenomenon.

★★★

If inspired technological advances and reasonable planet stewardship become pillars of the human condition, then thousands of new generations should have the environment and resources needed to flourish on earth.

★★★

The human condition has always been – and continues to be – fraught with angst. That's why spiritual teachers have, throughout the ages, urged their followers to be *in* the world, not *of* the world. That is to say, do not attach great importance to the world's ever-unfolding drama. And in a similar vein, it's wise to distance yourself from negativity.

★★★

Could it be that humanity's only crime is the pursuit of happiness? Isn't it starkly evident that people do what they *think* will bring them happiness? Of course, misguided choices lead to a broad range of outcomes, from harmless disappointments to stunning catastrophes. Still, there's often a lack of malice or harmful intent.

★★★

On some level, everyone in this world has chosen to be here – to learn and grow and savor and celebrate life, both its triumphs and its trials. Individuals, of course, have a wide range of needs, and life lessons unfold accordingly. For instance, some must learn how to be humble despite their vast wealth; while others must learn how to be noble despite their abject poverty.

★★★

Here's why you should be optimistic. The universe, the earth, and humanity's welfare are cradled in the arms of God – exactly where they need to be. It's up to a Higher Power to save life on earth. Therefore, place your trust in God; and rest easy.

★★★

Closing reflection ...

In his book *Enlightenment Now*, Harvard professor Steven Pinker uses statistics and graphs to prove that, around the world, violent crimes are declining; poverty is trending downward; wars are less frequent; people are living longer; wealth is expanding; literacy is rising; infant mortality rates are falling; and stunning technological advances in science, medicine, and industry are improving our quality of life. In other words, right now – despite the recent challenges of a pandemic – is the best time in history to be living on our planet! But those who only pay attention to social media, or to reports featured in national and global news, are completely unaware of this encouraging fact.

What does this mean to you?

★★★

As individuals expand their consciousness, they become more loving; and collectively, the world becomes a kinder, gentler place. But humanity's evolution doesn't stop there. As individuals grow in love, the stage is set for dramatic, global advances – for love is the *source* of insights, innovations, and breakthrough discoveries.

The quality of life for Americans has improved exponentially since our country's founding. Take a moment to reflect on just the past 75 years in the United States. Try to name five transformative inventions or discoveries that were made by U.S. citizens.

Finally, look at worldwide advances in technology over the last 25 years. How have they transformed your life at work and at home? Is there not clear evidence that love is flourishing?

★★★

DAY TWENTY-TWO

THE EPOCH OF BELIEF

> Creeds, traditions, morals, and ethics are ideological and behavioral norms transmitted by religious teachings, by example, and by word of mouth. They represent wisdom distilled through the ages. *Walter E. Williams*

★★★

Once again, why does a book on wellness and harmony include material on political, ideological, and sociological themes? Remember, your perspective of the world – be it positive or negative – ultimately affects your attitude at home and at work. It might be a subtle, unconscious influence, but the effect is real nonetheless. So take a moment to reflect on the following …

GEOPOLITICS

For thousands of years – and in all parts of the world – tribes and nations have fought one another for the right to occupy prized regions of land and, of course, to benefit from the resources and advantages tied to that land. Fierce battles were commonplace, and those who triumphed expanded their borders. Similar confrontations are prevalent today. Around the globe, strategic expanses of rich land and teeming water have changed hands countless times.

★★★

Historically, borders have unified a nation's people by promoting allegiance, pride, and a common identity. Riots and violent civil disturbances are fueled by feelings of bitterness, anger, and victimization. Indeed, highly charged emotions can obscure the bonds and commonalities that would normally unite a country's populace.

★★★

The rise and fall of nations and empires have much in common with the beginning and ending of personal relationships. As soon as oppression and exploitation become the norm, decline has already started. At the moment holiness, respect, and concepts of right and wrong are cast aside, dissolution has already begun – for such choices defy God's will.

★★★

It must be disheartening to witness the demise of an accomplished civilization. Yet, God's plan for humanity rises above the transient nature of governments and hierarchies. All that's needed is someplace where people can live freely, work harmoniously, and care for one another.

★★★

There have always been deranged leaders who desired to either conquer or destroy humanity. Typically, such individuals plotted under the guise of a cause, a political movement, or a religion. And throughout the ages, these psychopaths have been removed from society. They've been defeated, imprisoned, exiled, or executed; for megalomania and a thirst for martyrdom are difficult to cure – and the afflicted seldom recognize their need for help.

★★★

Pause to reflect on this historical overview which compares socialism to capitalism.

Socialism *vs.* Capitalism is …

- Controlled planning *vs.* Creative problem solving
- Predictable results *vs.* Surprise outcomes
- Using standard methods *vs.* Developing better ways
- Ideology and dogma *vs.* Knowledge and information
- Regulated markets *vs.* Free markets
- Rationing resources *vs.* Expanding resources
- Directives *vs.* Discussions
- Redistributing wealth *vs.* Building wealth
- Consolidating power *vs.* Sharing power
- Unaccountable central government *vs.* Responsive local government
- Reliance *vs.* Self-Reliance
- Tyranny *vs.* Liberty

Free markets promote affordable prices and also elevate the quality of goods and services. Therefore, the poor and disadvantaged benefit from a free market economy more so than any other demographic.

★★★

What is driving our bold new advances in medicine, manufacturing, agriculture, and technology? Quite simply, it's the incentive of making a profit. That's why virtually all breakthroughs – major discoveries that elevate humanity by improving our quality of life – occur within nations that promote free markets. Though love is the *source* of such advances, profit is the motivation.

★★★

As the world turns ...

- Misguided politicians enact flawed policies.
- Flawed policies expand human suffering.
- The people entrust politicians to alleviate human suffering.
- Politicians gain more authority and control over the people.
- Misguided politicians enact flawed policies.
- Flawed policies expand human suffering.

And so it goes.

★★★

Socialism is an economic ideology that serves as a stepping-stone to the economic and political ideals of communism. For decades, religious freedom and human rights have been scorned in socialist and communist nations, and state-enforced mandates have led to widespread human suffering.

★★★

At first, socialist countries are able to keep their promise of free everything for everyone. This is achieved by confiscating and redistributing privately held assets and property. But after businesses and industries are owned or managed by a central government, there's one outcome you can count on: an abysmal economy.

In the end, socialist countries are forced to stop giving things away. Why? It's because giveaways are not sustainable. Government leaders eventually run out of other people's money to spend. And when bankrupt countries carry on by simply printing more currency, their new money has very little purchasing power in the world market. The result is an economic deficit which triggers critical shortages and hyperinflation. Politicians, at that point, have no choice but to turn against the same people they promised to help. Then, instability opens the door for a dictator to seize control.

***

Socialism is rooted in good intentions, and it paints a utopian picture: Everyone will be equal; there will be no winners or losers; everyone will get along; no one will be poor or ridiculed; no one will be hungry or homeless or bullied; and so on. Yet in practice, true socialism has *never* brought lasting prosperity to the masses.

***

One can argue that America's rule of law, the judicial arbiter of every U.S. citizen, is ultimately tied to the worldviews and religious beliefs of our nation's founders. Both Judaism and Christianity embrace the first five books of the Old Testament, which is where you will find the Ten Commandments: God's directives on worship and moral behavior. Now fast-forward to the early 1940s, when politicians began using the phrase "Judeo-Christian ethics" as a way to unify Americans. Fully aware of this trend, President Franklin Roosevelt, at the start of the Second World War, urged men and women to "defend not just their homes, but their tenets of faith and humanity." Later still, the term "Judeo-Christian values" gained popularity, and President Lyndon Johnson referenced it while promoting civil rights legislation in the 1960s.

***

America's rule of law is built upon presumed innocence. This means a citizen is legally innocent until allowable evidence is presented to a jury of peers, and the jury reaches a guilty verdict. No one ever has to prove his or her innocence. To the contrary, prosecutors bear the burden of proving guilt.

***

America is not without problems. Yet, for those who value personal liberty and bountiful opportunity, there isn't a better place to live. Just know that equal opportunity doesn't lead to equal outcomes.

★★★

Frederic Bastiat was a French economist, a renowned statesman, and a fierce defender of liberty. Following the revolution of 1848, France was in political turmoil, and socialism threatened the interests of its citizens. Bastiat understood that an expanding central government undermines the natural harmony of human interactions. He once asked, "Is there a greater evil than converting the law into an instrument of plunder?"

Bastiat observed that most people believe laws are written to guarantee justice. He noted, however, that this view isn't accurate. The real purpose of the law is to prevent injustice. Here, Bastiat is affirming justice as humanity's natural, God-ordained state; while injustice is a foreign, man-made construct. Or think of it this way: While liberty is power, law is force.

★★★

At any point in modern history, relatively few humans are enjoying the gift of unfettered liberty. All others are, to some degree, facing the threats of tyranny.

★★★

Political correctness suppresses free speech. But beyond that, political correctness enables favored ideas and ideals to become sacrosanct, thereby prohibiting normal, healthy discussions of opposing views.

★★★

Why do great tribes and nations disappear? The long list of reasons includes natural disasters, wars, invasions, genocide, disease, famine, the rejection of God, a deterioration of the rule of law, pervasive ignorance, and a breakdown of the family unit. Additionally, persecution and

185

corruption and immorality have triggered some of humanity's most dramatic downfalls. In other words, many of the greatest dynasties and empires collapsed under the weight of cruelty, greed, debauchery, and cultural decay. And because human tendencies are slow to change, history keeps repeating itself. Still, these forlorn destinies are not just wasted endings; they are new starts – fresh beginnings ripe with opportunity.

★★★

Let's be honest. Some of us are warriors, but most of us are worriers. We wrestle with big problems, and little ones. We struggle with real fears and imagined ones. Yet, much of what we worry about never actually happens. What's more, some of our greatest fears are tied to things we can't control – such as floods, droughts, hurricanes, tornadoes, wildfires, earthquakes, tsunamis, and so on. When it comes to things we can't prevent, is there ever a good reason to worry? Is there ever a benefit?

★★★

In today's world, virtually everything is politicized. And sadly, a disturbing number of politicians are more interested in accumulating power, control, and wealth than they are in serving the best interests of their respective countries. Ambitious government leaders who want to expand their power will often use a devious ploy: Scare the citizens. When doomsday scenarios are promoted – and when human tragedies are politicized – people are more willing to surrender personal liberties in exchange for a larger government that promises safety. But as political leaders gain additional power, some will become corrupt; some will betray the people who trusted them.

★★★

As commander-in-chief of the Union Army, Abraham Lincoln observed that most individuals are able to handle hardship; but if you want a true test of character, give a person power.

★★★

Judging and doubting are products of the mind, whereas knowing and trusting are matters of the heart. Your mind shouts, *I have an opinion on the world and everything in it. Listen to me!* All the while your heart gently whispers, *Turn inward when searching for truth and reality. Heed my advice.* You can only obey one master. So moving forward, whose guidance will you choose to follow? Whose voice will you honor and cherish?

★★★

Fear is the natural response to an inherent human trait: weakness. But here's a tip. The next time something frightens you, ask God to replace *your* weakness with *his* strength. The instant you do this, you have nothing to fear!

★★★

Only one thing rivals the heartbreak of a tragedy: the person who uses it to advance his own misguided agenda. Such a person desecrates the pain of those who are hurting.

★★★

God is the foundation of all truth and reality. Therefore, people who exclude Divinity from their worldview will inevitably make erroneous judgments that will lead to mistaken conclusions.

★★★

While freedom is God-given, liberty is granted by government. Freedom rests entirely within the boundaries of an individual, whereas liberty is either fostered or hindered by a nation's laws.

★★★

Democratic and representative governments need checks and balances, such as strict term limits and rigorous ethics monitoring. Without proper safeguards, even beneficent governments will eventually be plagued by systemic corruption.

★★★

Although life isn't fragile, civilization is. A nation that does not recognize the sanctity of human life is destined to wither.

★★★

Turning away from God brings added pain and suffering.

MORE ABOUT PAIN

There are different kinds of pain and, if it were possible, many of us would avoid each one of them. Yet, a closer look at human pain reveals some surprising benefits. For instance, physical pain is an alarm, a warning that signals a problem with your body. If not for pain, most injuries and diseases would go undetected and, therefore, untreated. And without treatment, a minor problem could become more serious, perhaps even life threatening. Though you may not welcome physical pain, you can be grateful for knowing that something is wrong. In this sense, pain is a helpful friend.

★★★

The clinical term is congenital analgesia, the inability to feel physical pain. It's a serious condition because experiencing pain is vital for human survival. Still, pain is drenched in irony. For pain can motivate people to make better choices that, in turn, lead to improved health; and pain can spark existential questions that nurture spiritual growth. But pain can also trigger despair, depression, and thoughts of self-harm.

★★★

Eckhart Tolle suggests that everyone carries a burden of emotional pain caused by past experiences. He calls it a "pain-body." Moreover, this pain-body is the source of your over-reaction to minor annoyances that occur all the time. However, by monitoring your emotions, you can identify the situations and disturbances that trigger intense episodes of sadness, anger, or fear. And here's the key. Once you're aware of these triggers, you can recognize the beginning of an exaggerated, emotional response. Then, you can pick an intervention – such as a deep breathing exercise – to prevent a small setback from becoming a total meltdown. To say it another way, you can choose to react differently.

★★★

Therapists advise that it's better to "lean into" your pain, rather than resist or deny it. What does this mean to you? How might you benefit by leaning into your pain?

★★★

Hospice patients commonly experience death anxiety, which typically results from fear, pain, or both. Fear is usually sparked by a fear of the unknown, a fear of Divine judgment, or a fear of losing personal control. As for pain, it is either physical, emotional, or spiritual – or a combination thereof.

Meds can effectively manage physical pain, but they do nothing for emotional or spiritual pain. A host of issues can lead to emotional pain, including unfinished business and damaged or estranged relationships. And spiritual pain may stem from issues tied to guilt, shame, unworthiness, hopelessness, or forgiveness. With so many variables in play, the source of death anxiety is difficult to pinpoint, especially when the patient is unable to communicate.

That's why effective hospice care requires an interdisciplinary team. This core group includes a physician and nurse to provide clinical care, a social worker or counselor to offer psychosocial support, and a chaplain to provide spiritual care. Optimal outcomes are best achieved by addressing the needs of body, mind, and spirit.

★★★

You know that your death is inevitable. But by God's grace, you don't know when it will happen.

RELIGION AND SPIRITUALITY

Our world has different religions, just as it has different languages, cultures, and traditions. Ultimately, religions serve as pathways that connect humanity to Divinity.

Theistic religion is defined as a set of beliefs linked to a deity-created universe. Religions usually include sacred texts, rituals, worship, devotions, celebrations, and moral codes. Each religion features treasured stories, and each story imparts an essential lesson. Often, these lessons teach followers how to live a meaningful, righteous, and holy life.

★★★

Spirituality centers on one's inner self, and embraces a host of diverse perspectives; but spirituality always includes an acceptance that we are part of something much bigger than ourselves.

Ideally, religious and spiritual people are striving to be kind, loving, and respectful; and they genuinely care about all life on earth.

In a perfect world, individuals on religious or spiritual journeys are growing more humble, balanced, and devoted. Hopefully, such motivated people are becoming more rooted in reality; they are striving to be the embodiment of perfection, and progress is measured by the amount of joy in their hearts.

★★★

Redemptive suffering is the Christian tenet that personal suffering, when accepted and offered in union with Christ's death on the cross, can atone for one's sins. Redemptive suffering, however, is not the same as forgiveness, which stems from God's grace and is freely given through Jesus.

★★★

The cross symbolizes both suffering and Divinity.

★★★

Humanity is governed by two sets of laws: laws crafted by men and women, and laws ordained by God. Even if a thief evades captivity, justice will be served. Even when a killer's identity remains unknown, justice will prevail – for nothing escapes God's awareness. Sometimes, the scales of justice are balanced in the here and now. Other times, such reckonings unfold in the afterlife.

★★★

In truth, your choices have very real consequences. It's how you learn. Greed or anger-driven interactions attract more of the same. On some occasions, you'll be the perpetrator. Other times, you'll be on the receiving end. Just realize that the subsequent consequences are actually self-inflicted.

★★★

When you're attempting to escape a cycle of destructive behavior, commit to making better choices. By design, kind and helpful interactions will attract more of the same.

★★★

Closing reflection ...

On the topic of Divine judgment, Catholic priest and theologian, Thomas Merton wrote: "Why should anyone be shattered by the thought of hell? It is not compulsory to go there. Those who suffer do so by their own choice, and against the will of God. They experience hell by defying and resisting all the work of Providence and grace. Ultimately, it is their own will that condemns them, not God's."

What does this mean to you?

★★★

DAY TWENTY-THREE

DIVINE ORDER

Whether life is ugly or beautiful, there is
Divine Order to it. *Isaiah Washington*

★★★

Divine Order is the foundation of our universe and the fabric of universal law. Current evidence indicates that universal laws govern both the unthinkably small and the unimaginably large. Physicists believe that the slightest variance in today's elegant, cosmic dance could lead to chaos. In other words, without structure and cohesiveness, life as we know it cannot exist. Yet, cosmologist Charles Hellaby posits that the foundational mathematics and physics of our universe existed *before* the Big Bang. Otherwise, the universe would have been chaotic and dysfunctional from the very beginning. Hellaby suggests that only two questions remain: How could universal laws exist before the beginning of time? And who created them?

Indeed, could an ever-expanding, interconnected cosmos exist without Divine Order? Is it likely that our universe – more precise than a Swiss watch and more harmonious than a concert piano – is random and rudderless? Is it possible for life to flourish without a Maker's watchful eye?

Divine Order, however, reaches far beyond physics; its dominion includes metaphysics as well. What's more, Divine Order is the backdrop of daily experiences and interactions. Here's how it works. First, bear in mind that you're a spiritual being on a human journey. So think about all the people who share the stage with you as life unfolds. The joys, the struggles, the triumphs, the tears – all of these are experienced with people who join you, and ultimately leave. Do they not come into your life at just the right time? Does life not offer perfect opportunities to learn and grow? And does life not afford chances to strengthen your relationship with God?

Fortunately, you can ease into the reality of Divine Order – and minimize your pain – by following a few rules.

1. Live your life in the present moment. This principle is the building block of inner peace.
2. Do not resist what *is*. Acceptance is a required component of spiritual equanimity.
3. Practice patience. Patience fosters calmness and serenity.
4. Be more trusting. Placing your trust in God promotes a sense of safety and well-being.
5. Grow in love. As your love grows, your faith will grow as well.

While these guidelines are easy to understand, they're difficult to integrate. Still, all you really need to do is relax and embrace life exactly as it comes to you. By making this choice, you can avoid fear and mitigate anger. You can respond to adversity in a manner that reflects your values. And you will feel empowered, not victimized.

★★★

Those who insist on judging things are only increasing their stress. Those who keep resisting reality are only increasing their fatigue. And those who choose to continually judge *and* resist are following a frustrating path that will lead to utter exhaustion.

★★★

A carcass provides nutrition for scavenging birds and animals. A rotting tree is the womb for new vegetation. And by design, plants breathe in what animals and humans breathe out. The circle of life and Divine Order are threads of the same tapestry.

★★★

Ultimately, love triumphs over evil; and life prevails over death.

★★★

There are no conflicts among Divine Order, universal laws, and scientific truth.

★★★

As a manifestation of God's love, organic life is resilient and tenacious beyond what we can imagine. Life on our planet can be attacked, but not crushed. It can be threatened, but not extinguished.

★★★

Naturalists have learned a great deal by observing the wolf packs that roam Yellowstone National Park. And as we study the behavior of animals, we often see interactions that are similar to our own. Alpha male wolves, for instance, project quiet confidence and self-assurance. They understand their role and know what's best for the pack. They lead by example, which has a calming affect on the other wolves. An alpha male isn't aggressive to pack members. He's emotionally secure, like a great champion who has nothing left to prove.

The most famous Yellowstone wolf led his pack for more than seven years. This "super wolf" was a fierce defender of his family. In fact, he never lost a fight with a rival male from another pack. The super wolf's pack was the largest and most prosperous of all. Yet, within his own family, he loved to wrestle with little pups, often letting them "win." The super wolf would spend extra time with undersized or frightened pups in order to build their confidence. This patriarch was strong, yet gentle and caring.

Fittingly, park rangers discovered that alpha females also have a leadership role in their pack. They make many of the decisions, including when to travel, when to rest, and where to hunt. As one Yellowstone biologist noted, "It's the alpha female who runs the show." And as for humans, more men should follow the path of Yellowstone's super wolf: to live with quiet confidence; to lead by example; to be devoted to family; to be helpful and respectful; and to share in family responsibilities.

Adapted from an article by Carl Safina

★★★

Nature is not only a showcase of beauty, it's a display of abundance!

★★★

Physics and mathematics can only take you so far on your quest for ultimate truth. Then, spiritual work will lead you to your final destination.

★★★

Stars, planets, and moons are, on one level, individual and independent. But on another level, they are wholly connected. Orbiting planets depend on a star's gravitational pull. For without this attraction, planets would travel randomly through space. Sooner or later, they would be destroyed. In a similar way, each moon relies on a planet's gravitational pull to maintain its unique orbital path. But that's not all. In order for a planet to support life, there must be a nearby star with the perfect ratio of mass, heat, and light. What's more, the planet itself has to have a protective, nurturing atmosphere. Our universe is, indeed, an elegant balance of dependence and independence.

As for humanity, individuals travel a unique path that is part of a collective journey. On one level, each man, woman, and child is separate. But on another level, humans are joined and connected. We rely on one another for help and support. Families share food, shelter, and resources. And we yearn for companionship and community. That's why humanity's survival – individually and collectively – is dependent on love.

★★★

Organic life offers countless examples of what scientists call "the rule of spontaneous order." It's the attraction that compels fish to swim in schools. It triggers insects to swarm in the air. And it prompts birds to migrate in flocks, and animals to travel in herds. This behavior promotes survival because there is, in fact, greater safety in numbers. However, spontaneous order is even more complex; for it includes an entire subset of rules.

Within a school of fish, for example, individuals maintain a distance of one body length from their neighbors. And within a flock of birds, individuals stay three to four body lengths apart from one another. These rules enable massive groups of fish and birds to execute breathtaking twists and turns in unison. Their fluid movements seem choreographed, not improvised. And these amazing formations – sculptures in motion – not only mesmerize human spectators, predators are too confused to capture a meal.

Remarkably, the rule of spontaneous order applies to mechanical objects as well – which explains, in part, why randomly started pendulum clocks will eventually synchronize. Attractions, vibrations, pulses, fields, grids, frequencies, rules, and boundaries: all are invisible, yet undeniably real. In truth, they are the infrastructure of our universe.

★★★

Never forget that you are part of something much larger and greater than yourself.

★★★

On our planet, certain types of beetles are predators and certain varieties of trees are prey. Whenever a healthy tree is attacked by insects, the surrounding trees release a chemical designed to repel a similar attack. Has Mother Nature provided a way for trees to "talk" to one another?

★★★

To place one's trust in Divine Order is, in essence, a test of patience.

★★★

A smile crept across Jane's face as she read the invitation to her high school class reunion. *This will be fun*, she said to herself. But when Jane tried to book a flight, there was nothing available for that weekend. Lamenting her bad luck, she decided to drive to the reunion – an eight hundred mile round trip. Half way to her destination, Jane had another setback: steam began rising from the hood of her car. A wrecker towed the ailing Honda to a nearby dealership. Tears formed in Jane's eyes as Jeff, the service manager, introduced himself. After listening to her dilemma, Jeff sprang into action. He offered Jane a loaner car so that she could make it to the class reunion. Finally, Jeff promised that her Honda would be fixed by the time she returned to the dealership. Jane thought, *What a nice guy!* In the end, this unlikely encounter proved to be life-changing: For Jane had just met the man she would marry!

★★★

Examine your own life experiences. Can you recall any situations that were upsetting or annoying, but turned out to be blessings in disguise?

★★★

Resisting what you cannot change will spark anger and anxiety. Eventually, such resistance brings fatigue and depletion.

★★★

Although you cannot alter the past, your moment by moment choices *will* change the future. Today's empowering choices set the stage for tomorrow's fulfilling journey.

★★★

Eastern mystics teach that what we've done in the past determines the circumstances we face in the present. Yet karma is an active process, so we are not destined to be victims. The initiatives we take now will shape our future. And because each day's choices make a difference, we are never helpless or hopeless. Ultimately, karma provides opportunities to make amends; and by making amends, we begin to heal. Western theology, coincidentally, has its own version of karma: You reap what you sow.

★★★

There's a high probability that before the immense expansion had begun – before the Big Bang – an enormous and equally powerful compression had occurred. Therefore, structural and foundational components existed prior to the birth of our universe and the beginning of time. And it's quite likely that a boundless consciousness was part of that primordial mix as well. So is it rational to assign a name to this celestial essence which preceded life as we know it? Is it reasonable to call it God?

★★★

Natural creations evolve in dynamic, but predictable, cycles of expansion and compression: the beginning and ending of a flower, a bird, a star, or a universe – as if God were breathing in and breathing out.

★★★

Periods of expansion and compression are found *within* life cycles as well. Young people, for instance, are collecting and accumulating, while older people are simplifying and downsizing. And people who live or work in crowded, urban environments often choose to vacation or spend their weekends in the expanse of the countryside.

★★★

In physical domains, energy is the eternal power which fuels life; however, spirit *is* life. By its nature, spirit is also eternal. Moreover, spirit is at home in both physical *and* metaphysical realms.

★★★

Sometimes, the chicken precedes the egg. Other times, the egg precedes the chicken. It all depends on when the passerby arrives. Yet, each traveler is accompanied by a presence that remains constant and unchanged: the Creator of both the chicken *and* the egg.

★★★

On our planet, Divine Order includes a season of decline that culminates in death.

★★★

Closing Reflection ...

As a hospice caregiver, you have both a conscious and unconscious awareness of death. Sometimes, the death of a patient, a friend, or a family member will trigger thoughts of one's own mortality. Has this happened to you? Have you ever paused to reflect on the certainty of your death?

★★★

The following exercise is recommended by author and motivational expert, Steve Chandler. While this contemplation is amazingly therapeutic, it requires a great deal of introspection and courage. If you're uncomfortable — at any time, or for any reason — simply stop. You can always revisit this exercise another day ...

Find a private and quiet place, and imagine lying on your own deathbed. Close your eyes and think about saying your final goodbyes. In your mind, identify the people who have significantly impacted your life – those who have either helped or harmed you the most. Now, invite these people to your bedside, one at a time. Speak out loud to each person. This is the last chance to share your feelings with these individuals, so leave nothing unsaid. This is *your* goodbye, *your* journey. No one is judging you. There are no right or wrong things to say, and there are no right or wrong feelings to experience.

★★★

DAY TWENTY-FOUR

COURAGE AND EXCEPTIONALISM

> Success is not final, and failure is not fatal: It is the
> courage to continue that counts. *Winston Churchill*

★★★

Collectively, the human experience offers lots of opportunities for people to face hardship and to emerge victorious. Much of the time, our trials and troubles are minor and ordinary. But human beings can, when necessary, summon remarkable courage and strength; and in doing so, they are able to confront and overcome extraordinary circumstances. By our nature, we're fascinated by exceptional triumphs. Such stories trigger thoughts of awe. And they also spark soul-searching questions, like: *Could I endure something like this? Would I be able to bear such pain?* Perhaps the following story will evoke a similar kind of reflection.

Navy gunner Donald Stratton awoke Sunday morning at his normal time, expecting a routine day. A nearby calendar announced the date: December 7, 1941. Stratton climbed a ladder and stood on the sun-drenched deck of his current home, the U.S. Navy battleship, *Arizona*. Before long, he heard the faint drone of aircraft engines and what sounded like muffled explosions. Suddenly, the ship's air defense alarm sounded, followed by an order to "Man your battle stations!" Stratton dashed up a ladder to the radio shack, climbed another ladder to the signal bridge, took a third ladder to the main bridge, and raced up a fourth ladder to his assigned station, the sky control room. Within minutes, it seemed like all of Pearl Harbor was in flames, and the noise was deafening.

By now, five more sailors had joined Stratton inside the steel enclosure that housed an arsenal of antiaircraft guns. But with Japanese bombers flying underneath the range of the ship's guns, the *Arizona* was defenseless. Stratton and his crewmates watched in horror as the *Tennessee* and the *West Virginia* were pummeled. They witnessed the *Oklahoma* roll over and sink. And they saw nothing but a fireball where the *Pennsylvania* once stood. The Japanese planes were so low and so close to the ship, Stratton could see the face of each pilot. The *Arizona* took hit after hit. Thick black smoke billowed upward, and the air was saturated by the stench of burning fuel and exploding gunpowder.

Flames licked the walls of the control room; and the metal floor was so hot, the soles of Stratton's shoes began to melt. The crewmen knew they would die if they didn't leave their station soon. One at a time, the six men crept to the outside platform. For the moment, they were safe from the intense heat. But the crew – perched in an open space – was more vulnerable to the enemy's bombs and machine guns. Stratton paused to look at himself. Later, he recalled, "My legs were burned from ankle to thigh; and my shirt had caught fire, burning my chest and blistering my arms."

Then, a miracle began to unfold. Here's how Stratton remembers it:

"A breeze parted the smoke, and I saw a deckhand standing on an escort ship about twenty-five yards away. I motioned for him to throw us a rope. His first two attempts fell short. But on the third try, I tracked the rope as it sailed my direction, and I grabbed it in midair. Both ends were quickly anchored; so now, a lifeline bridged the seventy-five feet between our two ships. Still, our only hope was to dangle from a rope and travel the entire distance hand over hand, four stories above a raging sea. And as an added risk, most of us had severely burned fingers and palms. This would make the journey extremely painful, if not impossible.

"I shouted encouragement as, one by one, my five crewmates made it across safely. Finally, it was my turn. I had hardly started, and already I was feeling heat from the burning fuel below me. With a surge of adrenaline, I kept going. Maybe I thought I'd be letting the other men down if I gave up. The pain was excruciating, but I inched forward until, at last, the sailor from the escort ship snatched me from the air. I couldn't believe that we all made it – that no one had fallen or had been killed by the rain of machine gun bullets. We had help from the good Lord, I'm sure of that."

With burns covering sixty-five percent of his body, Donald Stratton's physical rehabilitation lasted more than ten months, and his mental and emotional healing took even longer. He had an incredible will to live, and was equally determined to fully recover from his injuries. Stratton was medically discharged from the Navy. But before the war ended, he re-enlisted and served once again in the Pacific Theater. The Pearl Harbor attack killed 2,403 Americans, and another 1,168 sailors and marines were wounded. A total of eighteen ships were sunk, including five battleships. Of the 1,511 crewmen assigned to the *Arizona*, only 334 survived.

Adapted from *All the Gallant Men* by Ken Gire

★★★

Those who achieve what others say cannot be done, never pay attention to such limitations again. *James Cook*

★★★

People who achieve great things have learned how to overcome adversity and failure. With that in mind, meet Temple Grandin. She was born in Boston on August 29, 1947 to successful and wealthy parents, Richard and Anna Grandin. But Temple's early childhood was far from normal. At six months old, she started to stiffen in her mother's arms. At ten months old, when people held her, Temple would scratch and claw them "like a trapped animal." Her world was one of heightened, amplified sensations which often left her feeling overwhelmed.

Temple showed a keen interest in odors and had a remarkable sense of smell. Her behavior was driven by sudden impulses, and she reacted bitterly when adults interfered with her self-assigned tasks. She knew nothing of the usual rules and conduct of human relationships. Temple recalls, "Normal children use clay for modeling; I used my feces and then spread these creations all over the room. I chewed up puzzles and spit the cardboard out on the floor. I had a violent temper, and when thwarted, I'd throw anything in reach – a museum quality vase, or maybe some leftover feces. I screamed almost continuously."

Yet, she also developed an immense power of concentration. Her attention grew so intense that she could create an orderly space of her own, a place of calmness in an otherwise chaotic world: "I could sit on the beach for hours sifting sand through my fingers and sculpting miniature mountains. I examined each grain of sand as though I were a scientist peering through a microscope. Other times, I studied the lines on my fingers, following each one as if it were a road on a map." By her third birthday, Temple was not yet talking. Anna found a speech therapist to work with Temple, and hired a nanny to play educational games with her.

Temple was evaluated by a special needs expert at Boston Children's Hospital and instead of being institutionalized – the most common choice of that era – she was enrolled in an exclusive, private kindergarten. Slowly but surely, Temple acquired the language skills needed to be a "high-functioning" adult on the autism spectrum. Then, by gathering courage and resolve, and by overcoming incredible odds, Temple attended college. She went on to earn an undergraduate degree in psychology, a graduate degree in animal science, and finally a PhD in animal science.

Like many autistic children, everything was literal to Temple. As a teenager, she listened to a minister read John 10:9 – "I am the door; whoever enters through me will be saved." Then, the preacher added, "Before each of you, there is a door that's opening to heaven. Find it and be saved." Temple would later write: "My mind centered on one thing – a door that opened to heaven. I had to find that door. I knew it wasn't the closet door, the bathroom door, the front door, or the door to the stable. Then one day I came upon a building I hadn't seen before. I went inside and climbed the stairs to the very top. And there it was, a small wooden door that opened onto the roof! A feeling of relief washed over me, a feeling of love and joy. I had found my door to heaven!"

Temple's contributions to the book *Beef Cattle Behaviors, Handling, and Facilities Design* revolutionized the complex operations of ranches, feedlots, and slaughterhouses worldwide. Grandin had always been okay with breeding, raising, and harvesting cattle for their meat. Her primary goal was to have calm, happy cows that were treated humanely. She worked to remove anything that might frighten or stress the animals, so that they could go gently and unknowingly to their death. The meat industry's goals were to increase productivity and process great tasting beef. As it happens, a happy cow moves more quickly and smoothly through the gates and chutes, thereby improving efficiency. And a calm cow doesn't release the stress hormones which taint the flavor of the meat. Because the beef from a happy, calm cow – one that is slaughtered humanely – tastes better and costs a bit less, Grandin's innovations were welcomed by meat processors.

Grandin points out, "Cattle are disturbed by the same kinds of sounds as autistic people: hissing air, high-pitched sounds, and sudden loud noises. But they are not bothered by low-pitched, rumbling noises.

Cattle are also agitated by high visual contrasts, shadows, and sudden movements. A light touch frightens them, but a firm touch calms them. I used to pull away from being touched, just like a wild cow. Gradually, I got used to being touched in a slow but firm manner, the same method that's needed to tame cattle." In terms of basic sensations and feelings, Grandin's shared experiences with farm animals compelled her to be sensitive to the needs of all animals and to advocate for their humane treatment. She became aware of these things through her own autism and, in part, because she had spent much of her childhood on farms.

Grandin believes that, when properly performed, slaughter is more humane than nature: "Just seconds after a slaughtered animal's throat is cut, endorphins are released and the animal dies calmly and without pain. When a sheep is attacked by a wolf, endorphins mitigate the pain as well — but only after the sheep has been terrified." It seems that Grandin's deepest feelings are for cattle; she feels a tenderness, a compassion for them that is intimate and very close to love. That's why she teaches people how to hold and handle cattle in the chute, how to transmit calmness to the animals, and how to bring them peace in the last minutes of their lives. For her, the lessons are half physical and half spiritual. Indeed, there is something very sacred in cradling an animal as it takes its final breath.

Because of her autism, Grandin thinks visually, not cognitively: "If you're a visual thinker, it's easier to identify with animals. If all your thought processes are in language, you can't imagine how cattle think. But if you think in pictures, it's much easier." She was shocked to learn that her notable power of visual imagery was not an attribute shared by everyone. Grandin is quick to mention that visual thinking is not, in itself, abnormal. She knows several non-autistic engineers who are able to "see" what they need to accomplish, make designs in their mind, and test them in imaginary simulations, just as she does.

Grandin's achievements have surpassed all expectations, and she has helped erase the stigma associated with autism as well. Temple is a professor at Colorado State University and a prolific writer. She's an expert on animal behavior and an international consultant on livestock care and management. Her autobiography *Emergence: Labeled Autistic* has become a must read for parents who have an autistic child. Sometimes, adults with autism and parents of autistic children are angry about this perplexing disorder. They may ask why people have to confront such difficult challenges. Yet, in Temple Grandin's case, if autism didn't exist, would there not be a troubling loss: a missing perspective on our interactions with animals?

Adapted from an interview by Dr. Oliver Sacks

Temple Grandin: Thoughts and reflections ...

I can remember the frustration of not being able to talk. I knew what I wanted to say; but I couldn't get the words out, so I would just scream.

There needs to be a lot more emphasis on what children *can* do instead of what they can't do.

When I'm with a cow, it's not a cognitive experience at all. I know what the cow is feeling.

The world needs different kinds of minds working together.

When I first held a cow, I thought, *What's happening to me?* I wondered if this was what love is.

If I could snap my fingers and be non-autistic, I would not – because I wouldn't be me. Autism is part of who I am.

The Rocky Mountains are pretty, but they don't give me a special feeling. When I look up at the stars at night, I know they are sublime, but I don't sense it. I would like to.

I can understand things intellectually. I sometimes think about the origin of the universe and why we are here.

Most people can pass on their genes. I can pass on my thoughts by writing books.

I want to do something important. I'm not interested in power or piles of money. I want to leave something behind. I want to make a positive contribution and to know that my life matters. These things are at the very core of my existence.

★★★

Closing reflection …

Think back on the lives and journeys of some of the patients you've served. Have there not been many who, in their own way, were courageous? Have there not been some who had shining moments of exceptionalism?

In your work as a hospice caregiver, have you ever had to "dig deep" for an added measure of courage? When facing complicated bedside care, how do you cope and persevere? What helps you stay calm and focused? How might such challenges help you become an even better caregiver?

Is it likely that a number of your patients have seen you as an example of exceptionalism? Could it be that your only limitations are the ones you place on yourself?

★★★

DAY TWENTY-FIVE

LAUGHTER

The most wasted of all days is one without laughter. *E. E. Cummings*

★★★

You were born with the gift of laughter. But did you know that laughter has therapeutic value? It lifts your spirits, lightens your mood, and makes you feel happier. Laughter also brings people closer together. It helps people feel more alive and empowered, and it promotes emotional and physical healing. In other words, laughing out loud is good for you! And as a result, a new health and wellness intervention has emerged: laughter therapy.

Laughter therapy uses humor to achieve improved health. More specifically, it allows the natural, physiological process of laughter to relieve stress. Laughter also helps you feel better about yourself and the world around you. Plus, it's a natural diversion – while laughing, your mind is free of all thoughts. What's more, laughter induces positive physical and chemical changes in your body. Studies have shown that laughing for just a few minutes can make you feel better for hours.

Why does it pay to laugh? Research has revealed that laughter:

- Exercises your heart and lungs
- Strengthens diaphragm and abdominal muscles
- Enhances oxygen intake
- Relaxes muscles and eases tension
- Triggers the release of endorphins
- Helps digestion
- Lowers blood pressure
- Improves your mental alertness
- Burns a few calories
- Boosts your immune system

Evidence suggests that laughter therapy may also:

- Improve your attitude
- Reduce stress, anxiety, and inflammation
- Stabilize blood glucose levels
- Improve sleep
- Enhance your overall quality of life
- Strengthen relationships
- Promote a general sense of well-being

★★★

Laughter is a wonderful door-opener for new relationships. It eases tension and builds trust.

★★★

Laughter is an ideal first-step to forgiving others and oneself.

★★★

Humor's origin is Divine.

★★★

Laughter cleanses the soul.

★★★

As it happens, the best humor always contains an element of truth.

★★★

Laughter diffuses tension and, therefore, promotes healing and well-being for individuals and relationships alike.

★★★

More on laughter ...

A good laugh heals a lot of hurts. *Madeleine L'Engle*

Laughter is sunshine in the house. *William Thackeray*

A smile is a curve that sets everything straight. *Phyllis Diller*

Always laugh when you can. It's cheap medicine. *Lord Byron*

Earth laughs in flowers. *Ralph Waldo Emerson*

He who makes his companion laugh deserves paradise. *Qur'an*

While laughter may not solve a problem, it will certainly dissolve a problem. *Madan Kataria*

If you don't learn to laugh at trouble, you won't have anything to laugh at when you're old. *Edgar Watson Howe*

Laughter is the most reliable gauge of human nature. *Feodor Dostoyevsky*

It's bad to suppress laughter. It goes down and spreads to your hips. *Fred Allen*

Laugh at yourself first, before anyone else can. *Elsa Maxwell*

Laughter has no foreign accent. *Paul Lowney*

★★★

Quantum physics includes something called the Many Worlds Theory. Here's a brief overview. As you face each fork in the road of life (and you make countless choices every day), part of you (an unconscious part) actually travels the path that you *didn't* take. These theoretical experiences unfold among an infinite number of parallel universes. So in another world, you filled up the tank *before* your car ran out of gas. In another world, you remembered to set the alarm, and you got to your team meeting *on time*. In a parallel universe, you said *Yes* to that blind date opportunity when you were a sophomore. And in a parallel universe, you passed your CHPN exam on the *first* attempt. The takeaway: Though life is always sacred, it isn't always serious.

★★★

Those who are wise have learned that laughter is healing. Like a soothing elixir, laughter eases stress. Like a loyal friend, laughter helps you cope with anxiety. Keep looking for opportunities to laugh!

★★★

After inviting God to dinner, the ego took its rightful seat at the head of the table.

★★★

Closing reflection ...

Can you recall an occasion when you started laughing and couldn't stop? Try to describe that feeling. And when your laughter finally subsided, how did you feel then? Were your sensations mostly pleasant? Would you like to experience those feelings more often? If so, how might that be achieved?

★★★

Always remember the distinction between laughing with someone, and laughing at someone.

★★★

Set aside one or two hours for watching a favorite comedy or comedian – something that you know will prompt laughter.

★★★

DAY TWENTY-SIX

WORK EXCELLENCE

Enlightenment is seeing God's love in all
that you encounter. *Jon Mundy*

★★★

In addition to being negative, many of our thoughts are simply not based in reality. The human mind tends to fabricate worst-case scenarios that rarely occur. Here's an example. Karen is a wonderful nurse. She's appreciated by patients, teammates, and management. Because of an unexpected problem at home, Karen reaches out to her supervisor, Linda. Karen writes an email requesting PTO for the following day. She provides an explanation for the short notice, and presses the "send" button at 9:00AM. By 11:00AM, Karen has already checked her email several times. There's been no response, and she's getting nervous. Karen thinks, *Linda should have got back to me by now. I wonder what's wrong?* At 1:00PM, there is still no response. Karen thinks, *This isn't fair. I do my best every shift, and I really need tomorrow off. Linda doesn't understand how important this is.* By 3:00PM, Karen thinks, *Linda doesn't like me. If she liked me, she would have approved my PTO by now.* At 4:00PM, there's a huge knot in Karen's stomach. She wonders, *Is Linda going to fire me? I really don't want to look for another job. This is terrible!* Karen checks her email at 4:30PM and learns that Linda has approved the PTO request. In her response, Linda apologized for not answering sooner; she was busy handling an urgent call for help. Alas, all is well – except for Karen's inner peace. She needlessly worried and stressed herself to the point of feeling sick.

★★★

Just as an ocean forms waves, the human mind forms thoughts. And much like waves, most thoughts are harmless. Yet a single, fictitious thought – when cultivated – can disrupt an entire day.

HOW TO EXCEL AT WORK

While most people want to be successful in their chosen career, many of us are unsure how to develop the attributes that are valued by employers – qualities such as keeping a positive attitude, acting in a professional manner, and being a team player. Human resource expert, Randall Hansen has addressed this need by offering some tips on how to excel at work. Here's a look at Hansen's insights ...

1. **Become an expert at doing your job.** Take pride in your work, and make the extra effort needed to erase any deficiencies. This will help you shine and stand out in a crowd.

2. **Develop a strong work ethic.** It isn't enough just to show up for work. Make sure you arrive on time, and don't leave early. Also, keep personal calls and distractions to a minimum.

3. **Strive to be professional.** Stay focused on your work. Professionals follow the rules, and they are courteous, helpful, and tactful. Professionals also look and dress appropriately.

4. **Demonstrate a positive attitude.** Nobody wants to be around a "Debbie Downer." So strive to have a positive, upbeat, can-do disposition. This appeals to coworkers and managers alike.

5. **Show initiative.** Look for better ways to do your job – new innovations that improve efficiency. Then, share these ideas with your supervisor.

6. **Be a team player.** Take a close look at how you interact with others. For a reality check, you might ask a teammate for honest feedback on how you might improve in this crucial area.

7. **Know your manager.** While you don't have to be a best friend, you do need to know your manager's expectations. By understanding those demands, you are prepared to meet them.

8. **Understand your employer's mission.** Make sure you know your employer's services and goals. This helps you understand your own role, as well as the value that you are adding.

9. **Be receptive to constructive criticism.** Yes, some supervisors are nitpickers, but most are simply offering ideas that will help you perform better. Welcome their advice accordingly.

10. **Cultivate new relationships.** Friendships in the workplace typically increase motivation and job satisfaction. Just be sure that your friends are as focused on work as you are.

11. **Accept opportunities to learn new skills.** Taking on new challenges will keep you from getting bored. Therefore, jump at those chances to improve existing skills and learn new ones.

12. **Be part of the solution.** Instead of just pointing out problems, be the person who finds clever solutions to them. Problem solvers are valued by every employer.

13. **Avoid gossip.** No matter how good you are at your job, getting caught in a web of rumors and gossip will quickly diminish your credibility in the workplace.

14. **Volunteer for new projects.** Not only will you score some points with your manager, new responsibilities can lead to more skills, better performance, or even a new career direction.

15. **Mentor new employees.** This can be a highly rewarding assignment. You help shape the talents of a new hire, and gain the appreciation of management at the same time.

Hansen maintains that success isn't necessarily tied to impressing a supervisor or getting a promotion, it's more about experiencing a sense of accomplishment for a job well done. Remember that when you're new to a job, keep asking questions. It's better to ask more questions and thoroughly understand your tasks, rather than proceed blindly and stumble miserably.

★★★

Kindness is a universal language that's expressed by a warm smile and a heartfelt embrace. Kindness is choosing to be friendly, caring, respectful, genuine, and considerate. People may not remember what you say and do, but they will always remember how you make them feel.

★★★

Kindness can be cultivated and nurtured. Through practice, kindness can be your default response to any situation; it can be offered unconditionally to loved ones and strangers alike. As you extend kindness, your thoughts are more positive – and less focused on yourself. Kindness doesn't need to be earned, for it costs you nothing to give.

★★★

"No one has ever become poor by giving." *Anne Frank*

★★★

Rather than coercing or cajoling people to do things on your terms and your schedule; and instead of pushing or pulling at those aggravating situations that inevitably arise, try practicing patience. Bear in mind that patience isn't just about waiting, it's keeping a positive attitude while waiting. Greater patience leads to reduced stress and better decision-making. And yes, patience is an essential element of compassion. So make a point to have patience for others, and for yourself as well.

★★★

American psychologist, Abraham Maslow created a new branch of humanistic psychology. In short, Maslow determined that people are constantly working their way through a complex hierarchy of human needs. Those needs range from the basic (food and shelter) to the sublime (oneness and peace). Additionally, he was curious how certain individuals were able to reach the pinnacle of human achievement: self-actualization. Maslow defines self-actualization as attaining one's full potential, or true self. Ultimately, he found that people who were high achievers shared a number of common characteristics.

215

- *An efficient perception of reality.* Self-actualizers are able to judge situations correctly and honestly. They are very aware of fake or dishonest behavior.
- *A comfortable acceptance of self and others.* Self-actualizers accept the flaws of human nature. Moreover, the hypocrisy and contradictions of the human condition are observed with humor and tolerance.
- *A reliance on personal experience and judgment.* Self-actualizers are independent thinkers. They don't rely on culture or environment to form opinions and views.
- *Are spontaneous and natural.* Self-actualizers are true to themselves, rather than being what others want them to be.
- *Are task centered.* Self-actualizers are fulfilling a life mission, usually something that is beyond or outside of themselves.
- *Are autonomous.* Although self-actualizers respect authority, they are not reliant on external supervision or motivation. Resourceful and independent, they dislike micromanagement.
- *A continued renewal of appreciation.* Self-actualizers constantly see life's basic goodness. Each sunset or flower is experienced as if it were the first time. And there's also an innocence of vision, like that of an artist or child.
- *Have profound interpersonal relationships.* The interpersonal relationships of self-actualizers are distinguished by deep, loving bonds.
- *Are comfortable with solitude.* Despite their satisfying relationships, self-actualizers value solitude and are comfortable being alone.
- *A non-hostile sense of humor.* Self-actualizers frequently find humor in life, but not at the expense of someone's embarrassment or pain. And of course, there's an ability to laugh at oneself.
- *Have peak experiences.* Self-actualizers often experience feelings of peace, harmony, and deep meaning. They describe such events as being one with the universe, or as being embraced by the love of a Higher Power.

- *Are socially compassionate.* While self-actualizers do not internalize another person's pain, they are keenly aware of human suffering – and will take action to lessen it.
- *Have select friendships.* Self-actualizers tend to have several close friends rather than a large number of superficial relationships.

In summary, self-actualizers typically feel safe, calm, loved, fulfilled, and vibrantly alive.

★★★

When at work, give your employer and your patients 100%. They deserve it. When at home, give your partner and your family 100%. They deserve it. And during those private, alone times, give yourself 100%. You deserve it!

★★★

If anxiety is building over an approaching work-related event, let your mind create a vision of it – a picture in which you are calm, confident, and successful. In addition to easing your current anxiety, this intervention sets the stage for a positive outcome

★★★

In care giving situations, inspiration is often more effective than perspiration.

★★★

Hospice caregivers face inherent risks. The work can be traumatizing. Yet, beauty is sometimes found in the pain.

★★★

When you are truly present with someone – focused, and free of agendas – your presence is profoundly healing.

★★★

Wherever you find two or more people, you find problems. So with discord firmly entrenched in the human condition, conflict resolution skills are highly valued – both at work and at home. Let's look at six tips that may help everyone get along a little better.

1. *Give your full attention to the person or persons in your presence.* In a one-on-one or group conversation, you must actually listen to what others are saying. This is a simple task, but not an easy one. And it's yet another example of mindfulness promoting positive outcomes.

2. *Discuss only one thing at a time.* Suppose your patient, Mr. Jones isn't taking his scheduled meds. In addition, Mr. Jones gets out of bed without asking his daughter for assistance, and he seldom uses the oxygen recommended by his respiratory therapist. While it's fine to point out the benefits of supplemental oxygen and transfer assistance, Mr. Jones may respond more favorably if you focus on just *one* issue right now: taking his medicine as prescribed. This sets the stage for reaching an agreement that's suitable to both you and the patient.

3. *Talk about your feelings, not your opinions.* You may want to try this one at home. Let's say that whenever you ask your husband, Robert for help around the house, he gets defensive and an argument ensues. Rather than giving Robert your opinion – *You should help more often!* – you might say: "I'm worried because I can't possibly finish all of the household chores. Could we make a to-do list and divide the jobs in a way that's manageable for both of us?"

4. *Put yourself in the other person's shoes.* This approach is also called active listening, and it shows that you understand how someone else feels. It validates people and respects their point of view. In the case of your patient, Mr. Jones who is a fall risk, you could say: "I understand why you prefer to get out of bed without help. Your daughter's busy doing other things, and you don't want to inconvenience her. But you and your daughter will be happier if you don't fall and get hurt. Please ask her for help when you get out of bed. Both of you will be better off."

5. *Try something different.* This technique works best with family. First, reflect on your own tendencies when facing a conflict. Do you get angry right away? Do you take things personally? Are you sarcastic or patronizing? Do you raise your voice? Once you've identified your typical reactions to a confrontation, make a determined effort to "switch gears." By changing your usual behavior, you can avoid the established ruts in your relationships. And as loved ones witness your change, they may listen more carefully to what you are saying. So if you're usually quick to anger, stay calm. If you typically raise your voice, then lower it. If you like to use sarcasm, then hold your tongue. The goal is to create an environment for constructive conversation.

6. *Compromise can be a good thing.* First, let go of any belief that there must be a winner and a loser in order to resolve a conflict. This view is simply a misguided conclusion. Remember Mr. Jones, your patient who ignored the recommendations of his respiratory therapist? Suppose you've already explained the benefits of using supplemental oxygen, but Mr. Jones continues to disregard your education and advice. Maybe a compromise would prove helpful. A hypothetical opener could go something like: "I know that using oxygen all of the time can be a nuisance. How about using it after you've been up for a while, right after your daughter helps you get back in bed?" In this scenario, both the nurse and the patient are making a reasonable concession. It's a compromise that meets the needs of all parties, and everyone leaves the discussion feeling respected.

★★★

Closing Reflection ...

Is it okay for some conflicts to remain unresolved? Why or why not? How do you build relationships with coworkers and patients that are strong enough to withstand disagreement? How are you showing respect for different points of view? How might cultural influences or religious beliefs impact the choices made by your patients? As a caregiver, how can you get better at putting yourself in another person's shoes? Finally, is "compromise" appropriate for your care giving toolbox? Why or why not?

★★★

DAY TWENTY-SEVEN

LIFE EXCELLENCE

> The wildflowers that nobody notices at the edge of the road
> are saints looking up at the face of God. *Thomas Merton*

★★★

A strong marriage, like most important things in life, is achieved by working at it. Therefore, the couples that make an effort to keep their marital vows are richly rewarded. The couples that value and nurture their relationship will likely grow stronger with each passing year. So if you're in a committed relationship, you may want to try the following suggestions that are endorsed by marriage counselors.

- **Start each day with a hug.** Expressions of love are always good!
- **Create rituals.** Establish routines that promote quality time together, such as sharing morning coffee, or reserving Saturday as a date night.
- **Establish a daily chat.** Start by giving your spouse a compliment, something you appreciate. Ask your partner to share any troubles or concerns. Offer your own worries or requests in a nonjudgmental way. End by talking about a hope or dream that you have in common.

- **Make important decisions together.** While discussing the pros and cons of an important decision, be sure to ask, *Will this choice be good for our marriage?*
- **Wear your wedding ring.** It offers a visual reminder of your commitment.
- **Be accepting of differences.** So you hope to change your spouse. Really?
- **Be polite.** Are you more courteous to strangers?
- **Be gentle.** Harsh words are very painful.
- **Offer gifts.** Give your partner a thoughtful gift – when it isn't expected.
- **Smile often.** Remember how much that meant when you first met?
- **Give a back rub.** Perhaps the next time, you'll be on the receiving end.
- **Be a good listener.** Make eye contact and give your undivided attention.
- **Laugh together.** Find things that *both* of you can laugh about.
- **Offer caring touch.** A soft touch on the shoulder or cheek makes a connection.
- **Call your spouse.** When possible, check in during the day.
- **Hold hands.** You can be intimate while taking a walk or watching TV.
- **Look your best.** Attention to grooming and wardrobe show that you care.
- **Ask, *How can I help?*** Just doing simple things will be appreciated.
- **Apologize.** Healing begins with: *I'm sorry, please forgive me.*
- **Reminisce.** It's fun to talk about special times that were shared together.
- **Be realistic.** Partners shouldn't be expected to "complete" one another.
- **Watch a sunset together.** Revel in the beauty.
- **Say, *I love you.*** The three words everyone wants to hear.

- **Pray together.** Since marriage is a Covenant, ask for God's blessing and guidance.
- **End each day with a kiss.** Expressions of love are always good!

★★★

If there's one guaranteed way to have an unhappy relationship, it's when each partner is focused on winning arguments and gaining power. But when each individual puts his partner's needs before his own, the marriage is rewarding and harmonious. In these instances, personal satisfaction is achieved by pleasing one's partner. Such relationships are centered on kindness and thoughtfulness − not about who's right or wrong.

★★★

There's an old proverb that reads, "Friends are flowers in the garden of life." Indeed, a friend can listen to your worries and lift your spirits. A friend can ease your loneliness and guide you through a crisis. And yes, friends come in different varieties as well. There are close, lifelong friends of the heart; and there are casual, fleeting friends of the road. Yet, like garden flowers, friendships need to be nurtured in order to grow healthy and strong. Following a study of relationships, writer and entrepreneur, Alaia Williams offered some insights on how to strengthen your friendships.

- *Choose wisely.* Become friends with people who build you up, not wear you down. Choose friends who inspire you, not insult you. Although you can't choose your family, you *can* choose your friends.
- *Listen closely.* Be sure to ask follow-up questions, and then reply with a summary of what you've heard. Good friends are good listeners.
- *Respond carefully.* Think before you speak, especially if you're upset. This helps you avoid hurting someone's feelings. Moreover, thoughtful answers build trust.

- *Don't be just a fixer.* If a friend asks for your advice, then give it. Otherwise, allow people the time and space they need to process things and find their own solutions.
- *Play fair.* If you're always trying to "one-up" a friend, eventually he or she won't want to play with you anymore.
- *Be authentic.* Be honest and be yourself. If someone can't accept you for who you are, then developing a meaningful friendship is a long shot at best.
- *Communicate openly.* When you're talking with a friend, always be forthright. Avoid hidden agendas.
- *Offer respect.* While it's okay to disagree with someone's choice, respect your friend's right to make that choice – even if it could be a mistake.
- *Do unto others.* In short, be the kind of friend you want others to be for you.
- *Be empathetic.* Imagine what it might be like to walk a mile in their shoes.
- *Give compliments.* Demonstrate your thoughtfulness by complimenting an attribute you admire. Remember to congratulate a friend who has achieved a significant goal.
- *Express gratitude.* Don't keep your friends guessing. Let them know how much you value their friendship.
- *Admit and apologize.* After doing something wrong, admit it. Then mean it when you say, "I'm sorry."
- *Forgive and let go.* Did a friend do something that hurt you? Have you talked it through? Was an apology offered? Then let it go! Instead of living in the past, try making a fresh start.
- *Make time.* Show your friends that you want to be with them. Juggle your schedule in order to meet for lunch. Or if you're exceptionally busy, keep in touch with a quick call or text.
- *Celebrate common interests and special occasions.* Many friendships begin with a common thread – for instance, a shared hobby or a mutual love of books. Allow these commonalities to strengthen your friendship. Also, use a calendar to remember special dates, like birthdays.

- *Be a promise keeper.* When you make a commitment, do your best to keep it. However, if you do have to break a promise, it's better to say, "I can't see you tomorrow, but let's go to the park on Saturday."
- *Try something new.* When you and a friend fall into a rut, make a point to do something different. It's all about enjoying your friendship and having fun.
- *Seek balance.* At times, you will either be giving more or receiving more in a friendship. But ideally, the giving and receiving will reach a balance.
- *Give encouragement.* Motivation and affirmation are important. If a friend isn't in your corner, who is?
- *Be discreet.* Private conversations with friends are confidential. Don't share them.
- *Withhold judgment.* Friendships come and go for lots of reasons. Circumstances change. People grow and mature. Perhaps it's just time to move on, and that's okay.

★★★

In the morning, write a "to-do" list. That way, there's no need to memorize what you hope to get done as your day unfolds. In the evening, a mental "ta-dah" list celebrates the things you accomplished.

★★★

If you're interested in sharpening your parental skills, take a moment to review the following advice. Even if you're intuitively aware of these guidelines, it may prove helpful to reflect on them ...

- Shower your children with unconditional love.
- Allow them to make mistakes and to learn that poor choices have consequences.
- Forgive your children.
- Respect them and be kind to them.
- Be a thoughtful teacher and a helpful guide.

- Establish fair rules and clear boundaries; then, remember to enforce them.
- Be patient with your kids.
- Avoid comparing a child with his siblings or with other kids.
- Be a role model, especially on matters of faith and morality.
- Spend time with your children – and actually be *present* for them.
- Laugh and have fun with them.
- Celebrate their achievements. And when your kids are struggling, offer comfort, support, and encouragement.
- Remember that you're a parent, not a best friend.
- Avoid living vicariously through your children. It's *their* journey, so let them chart the course.
- As your children get older, give them more freedom. Hopefully, they will recognize an important connection: greater freedom brings greater responsibility.

These parenting standards are tough to achieve and maintain. So when you fall short, don't be too hard on yourself. Fortunately, kids are amazingly resilient. They can withstand parental faults and flaws.

★★★

When you are offended by what someone says or does, it might be that – unconsciously – you see a disturbing aspect of yourself in that person.

★★★

More on victimhood ...

Those who embrace victimhood have a built-in excuse to achieve very little in life. Victims are not accountable for their choices because they blame others for their circumstances. Typically, they carry a misguided sense of entitlement, and their lives lack meaning. A victim's mantra: *It's not my fault.*

Seeing oneself as a victim leads to a negative self-image. Such a person typically becomes self-centered and wallows in self-pity. There is no belief in self-determined achievement or self-reliance. A victim thinks his or her future lies in the hands of others. Finally, there's no awareness of being part of something larger than oneself.

★★★

Still, the victimhood trap isn't the only destructive identity hazard to avoid. For instance, those who carry guilt and shame end up living in a pit of despair. They struggle with feelings of unworthiness, and their sadness is expressed through laments like: *I don't deserve to be happy. God is punishing me. I'm not worthy of forgiveness. It's all my fault.*

★★★

Claiming to be a victim soothes your ego, but troubles your heart.

★★★

Much like forgiveness, patience is a gift that is given to oneself. Patience allows life to unfold at its own pace; and by practicing patience, you receive the blessing of peace.

Tip: As you experience something that triggers anger or frustration, try redirecting your attention to something more pleasant. If you're stuck in traffic, for example, listen to music – or test your skill at identifying the makes and models of nearby cars.

★★★

Instead of pouring your heart out on social media, try pouring your heart out to God – the only "Like" that really matters!

★★★

Closing reflection ...

Step One

Based on the material presented in this chapter, write down three changes you can make that will improve things at home.

Step Two

From that list of three changes you're willing to make at home, select the most important one.

Step Three

Now that you've identified the single most important change you can make at home, start making that change right now!

★★★

DAY TWENTY-EIGHT

PEER INSIGHTS, PART ONE

The following survey includes the perspectives of seasoned hospice caregivers, including nurses, nursing assistants, social workers, and chaplains.

QUESTION: Looking back on your first months as a hospice caregiver, what were your biggest challenges?

A SAMPLE OF RESPONSES

My first months were more than twenty years ago, but I remember them vividly. AIDS was a leading cause of death at that time. Many young men – including some fathers – were dying. Secret lives were being revealed, and there was enormous sorrow. It seemed as though patients and loved ones were carrying their pain alone … as though they felt undeserving of God's love. It was a fearful time, and I experienced profound sadness.

★★★

My biggest challenge was accurately interpreting the signs and symptoms of end-of-life, and how to explain them to family members.

★★★

I felt the need to answer questions that, in reality, couldn't be answered; and I felt the need to fix problems that actually couldn't be fixed.

★★★

It took a long time to sharpen my documenting and charting skills, and become familiar with Medicare and Joint Commission rules and regulations.

★★★

I struggled to find the right words to comfort and reassure my patients and families.

★★★

It was hard to educate patients and families who were in denial, or were anxious and angry and not yet ready for end-of-life discussions.

★★★

I didn't know what to say, what not to say, or when and how to say it. Some patients wanted as much information as I could possibly give them. But others didn't want me to talk about their disease or their decline at all.

★★★

At times, I felt completely overwhelmed by my caseload and everything that I was expected to do.

★★★

When a patient died, I reflected on the journey we had shared. I had grown close to many of them. They were precious people, and I was saddened by their passing. The sheer number of deaths — and the abrupt loss of so many relationships — depleted me.

★★★

I remember my work being so fast-paced. New admissions and deaths were blurred together. I could scarcely catch my breath.

★★★

I wasn't sure if unresponsive patients could hear and understand the people who might talk to them. Nonetheless, I decided to introduce myself to every patient — including those who were nonverbal. I explained why I was there and what I was going to do. I made sure to say, *Goodbye.* And at some point during my visit, I reassured them that they were safe, and they were loved. Now I'm certain that, on some level, I'm connecting with these patients in a meaningful way.

★★★

My biggest challenge was not knowing what to say to family members when a loved one was actively dying. Gradually, I gained skill and confidence in guiding people through end-of-life journeys.

★★★

QUESTION: How did you overcome your initial challenges?

A SAMPLE OF RESPONSES

I learned to observe and respect each patient's journey. I came to understand and accept that everyone has the right to self-determined, end-of-life care. It became a core value – not trying to change what was working for my patients, even when their choice was to suffer rather than to take pain medicine. I realized that God's grace can be experienced through his gift of free will.

★★★

Perseverance was key. I found the courage to keep asking questions and to continue learning.

★★★

Nearly every shift someone would ask me, *How much time does she have?* Sometimes, patients look like they're going to pass at any moment, yet they might live for several more days. I think God was reminding me that I have no authority in this matter. I've overcome my feeling of helplessness by realizing that such things are beyond my control.

★★★

I make a point to seek advice from colleagues. Now I'm comfortable answering a question with the words, *I don't know.* I've accepted that there are things I can't fix.

★★★

For me, experience has brought improved confidence.

★★★

I've learned to expect much longer conversations with patients and families. I also realize that education is repetitive and never-ending. Patience is so important! People always know when you're in a hurry to get to the next visit.

★★★

I discovered that deep breathing helps me stay calm and focused. So right before visiting a patient, I take a minute to prepare and center myself.

★★★

After a patient visit, I take a moment to reflect on how it turned out. Was I helpful? What could I have done differently? How can I make my next visit better?

★★★

I'm still trying to overcome certain challenges. For instance, if a friend or family member is diagnosed with cancer, I remind myself that a cure is always possible. When people get sick, it doesn't mean they will soon be reaching out to hospice. It doesn't necessarily mean they are going to die.

★★★

I've learned that it's okay to talk to my supervisor when I feel overwhelmed by caseload demands.

★★★

I know that my relationships with patients and families must always include a "goodbye." Relationships with my patients are meaningful, but it's a different kind of investment than what I make with my own family or with a lifelong friend.

★★★

I make each visit count. I'm aware that the first time I see a patient might be the last time I see him.

★★★

I've established emotional boundaries that separate my patient relationships from my personal ones.

★★★

I have learned to turn negatives into positives. If I've done my best to help someone prepare for death, I feel that I've fulfilled my purpose. When a patient dies, I don't see it as a personal failure.

★★★

I've overcome my challenges at work through prayer and persistence. I've taken time to reflect on my own life experiences, both as a nurse and as an end-of-life caregiver for my mother. My hospice work has added so much meaning and purpose to my life. I feel truly blessed!

★★★

QUESTION: How do you manage being so up-close and personal with pain, suffering, and death?

A SAMPLE OF RESPONSES

Suffering is a natural, multifaceted part of the human experience. Pain can bring out both the best and the worst in people. But either way, it's a necessary element of life. Suffering can draw people closer to God, and it offers caregivers an opportunity to be compassionate. I view death much the same as birth – a miraculous event and a new beginning. Whenever I feel threatened, I find peace and safety through prayer. My greatest gift as a nurse has been to serve the dying.

★★★

I accept that death is part of life. But I'm sad when someone young dies.

★★★

I find comfort through my faith. I pray on my way to work every morning. Even in the face of suffering and death, I feel blessed in the work that I do. Also, it really helps that I'm part of a great crew. We work as a team and shoulder the burden together. We support one another, and that makes everything easier!

★★★

I believe my work is a privilege. Every day I'm reminded about what is really important in life. But I do have to remember to separate work from home life. And I have to recognize when I need to take some time off.

★★★

It's a privilege to be at the bedside of someone who's dying. Usually I can manage physical symptoms with medication, and I have an interdisciplinary team to address emotional and spiritual needs. I'm grateful for that.

★★★

I try to care for my patients as if they were family. But at the same time, I'm careful to keep boundaries. My heart knows the difference between my patients and my family.

★★★

At the bedside, I try to detach myself while focusing on the immediate task at hand. Also, I'm a true believer in heaven. I know that someone's life doesn't end when the body dies. The soul goes on to a better place.

★★★

I value each opportunity to witness and possibly alleviate someone's pain. I learn from these experiences, and I try to put them into a larger context of eternity *vs.* the season of life I see now.

★★★

It's a privilege to be part of something so intimate as end-of-life care. It's also humbling, as I'm reminded every day of the gift of life. I've learned that I don't always have to manage things, just appreciate them.

★★★

Honestly, I couldn't do this work without having a deep faith. I celebrate death's deliverance from suffering, which in itself is very healing. And I don't judge the circumstances surrounding a patient's death. I remember a husband explaining that he had prayed three different ways for his wife. When she first became sick, he prayed for healing. When her illness grew worse, he prayed for the pain to go away. And when the pain became too much for her to bear, he prayed that God would take her.

★★★

I listen intently to what my patients tell me. I understand the power of being heard. It's uplifting and transforming!

★★★

My work at the bedside is a ministry, a calling. Whatever strength I need comes from God.

★★★

I see myself as a companion, and I encourage my patients to lean into their spiritual pain. That said, I can only support them. In the end, each patient must own his personal pain.

★★★

I focus on the good that comes from helping my patients. At the end of each day, I'm proud of what I've done.

★★★

I know that I'm making a huge difference by managing pain, by listening to a concern, and by offering a hug. And I know that I'm never alone in my work, that God is always with me.

★★★

QUESTION: How do you maintain a healthy work–life balance?

A SAMPLE OF RESPONSES

For me, harmony is a product of creativity. At home, I like gardening and working in the yard. I enjoy walking my dog and visiting family and friends. But I also spend time alone, a choice which leads to greater clarity. My journey unfolds through the choices I make.

★★★

I leave work at work, and at home I take naps!

★★★

On my days off, I spend time with my husband and kids. I also have lots of hobbies that I love.

★★★

I turn off my cell phone when I'm not working, and I take time off when family needs arise.

★★★

I'm lucky to have a super-supportive family. And when I'm at home, I always look for reasons to laugh!

★★★

I know that when I'm home, I need to focus on my family. So I use the drive home from work to regroup and be ready for whatever happens next. I want to give my family 100% when I'm with them.

★★★

I take a walk every morning. I love to read, host cookouts, and go shopping on days off.

★★★

I often find myself thinking about work during my time at home. It's an ongoing struggle. Spending time in nature is the best way for me to clear my head. I go to a place where I only hear the sounds of birds, animals, wind, and water.

★★★

I'm active in my church, and I really enjoy interactions with children. They make me laugh, and maybe they keep me from growing "old." I exercise. I take vacations. I love camping. I like to drive my convertible – the breeze is both cleansing and refreshing! And because I live in the country, I'm able to raise chickens.

★★★

I make sure to take vacations twice each year. Vacations nourish my soul!

★★★

I maintain a close, peer-to-peer relationship with another hospice worker. It really helps me share and process my feelings.

★★★

On my morning drive to work, I identify three things that I'm grateful for. That way, I start the day with a positive mindset. I rarely get discouraged because, as the day unfolds, I make a point to remind myself of my blessings. I keep fit by walking and bicycling.

★★★

When I'm not at work, I do things I truly enjoy. It sounds so simple, but sometimes it isn't easy to put yourself first.

★★★

I love to hike in the woods. And on days off, I try to get extra sleep. I like to meditate, and I relax by taking a bubble bath.

★★★

I literally expanded my horizons by taking flying lessons and earning a pilot's license!

★★★

CLIMBING A MOUNTAIN: A GUIDED IMAGERY

We sit together, the mountain and me, until
only the mountain remains. *Li Bai*

★★★

People of all eras and cultures have been attracted to mountains. Towering above everything else on our planet, their sheer size is imposing, yet inspirational. Mountains have an inherent holiness, which explains why so many spiritual leaders have actually journeyed to a mountaintop – to a sacred space where they could connect with Divinity. Immense and timeless, mountains embody both harmony and harshness, majesty and peril. Early humans perceived them as guardians and protectors; and even today, mountains symbolize dependability and permanence.

With such grand history as a backdrop, get ready to climb a mountain. And because this adventure will unfold within your mind, start by taking three deep breaths ...

Your journey begins, as it must, with a first step. You're walking in a field of tall, lush grass. An early morning sun pierces the bright blue sky, and a gentle breeze signals that all is well. Your stride is smooth and effortless. You wonder, *How long will the path be so easy?* In response, the trail quickly turns upward, and each step requires a bit more effort. The tall grass is yielding to groves of hardy bushes, and billowing clouds are dotting the sky. Now the trail is even steeper, and late morning brings gusty winds as well. With a chill in the air, you're thankful for the jacket that's keeping you warm.

It's midday, and rocky outcrops dominate the landscape. Some of these formations are jagged and barren, while others are weathered and adorned by lichen. Your breathing is labored, and each footstep requires added determination. Still, you know that great dreams — by their nature — are only realized through exceptional resolve and perseverance. Suddenly, the pathway vanishes. Your eyes widen as you see just one option: to climb skyward. The only way to reach the summit is to navigate a near-vertical ascent. You're aware of a troubling paradox: the mountain is completely harmless, but potentially lethal. Your mind races, *Is it possible? Can I actually do this?*

The mid-afternoon sky is slate gray, and cold air is numbing your fingers. Taking a deep breath, you cautiously raise your left arm and right leg. Thankfully, your outstretched hand and dangling foot find a safe place to rest. This first, vertical step is followed by a second and a third. While inching upward on this perilous cliff, your mind is laser-focused — void of all thoughts. There is only *now*. Each subsequent step is accompanied by yet another. You begin to trust the mountain. You start respecting the mountain. Then, you are *one* with it.

Rather than fight an imaginary enemy, you simply surrender. But your choice isn't a sign of weakness, it's an act of courage. It empowers you. Rather than deny the level of risk, you embrace it. You accept what *is*. Climbing higher, the temperature continues to drop. Your head is engulfed by a penetrating mist, and a strong wind stings your ears. Conditions are deteriorating. Nonetheless, you push on; for the summit is close now, just a little farther …

Finally, with an aching body and a pounding heart, you reach the top of the mountain. The early evening vista is mind-blowing. The sky is a canvas of pinks and purples, and you are in awe of God's creations. You whisper a prayer of gratitude. The summit is still, yet alive; it is silent, yet wise; it is humble, yet proud. From this lofty elevation, your worries are insignificant. Perched above the clouds, it's clear that you are part of something much greater than yourself. You realize that you're *in* the world, but not of it.

On the mountaintop, you stand alone – but are not alone. Indeed, you are profoundly connected to your Creator. It isn't an accident that you're standing at *this* pinnacle, at *this* moment. Nor is it by chance that you recognize a deep meaning to life. And through God's grace, you know that each pathway is holy, and every journey is sacred.

Inspired by Jon Kabat-Zinn

★★★

Closing reflection ...

An excursion to a mountaintop – an endeavor hindered by setbacks and exhaustion, yet punctuated by bursts of progress and euphoria – has much in common with a typical life journey. Many people experience a moment when fear is conquered by courage, when self-doubt is eased by newfound confidence, and when a persistent illusion is unmasked by a sudden insight. Many of us have periods of worry that are vanquished by faith; moments of despair mitigated by hope; outbreaks of pain allayed by healing; intervals of cynicism shattered by awe; stretches of malaise jolted by inspiration; times of confusion lifted by clarity; and seasons of sadness that slowly fade and, ultimately, are replaced by joyful tears.

★★★

DAY TWENTY-NINE

PEER INSIGHTS, PART TWO

The following survey includes the perspectives of seasoned hospice caregivers, including nurses, nursing assistants, social workers, and chaplains.

QUESTION: How do you maintain healthy boundaries between your patients and yourself?

A SAMPLE OF RESPONSES

My boundary is an invisible fence that protects me (on one side) and my patients (on the other side).

★★★

The interactions I have with patients and their families are finite. When my shift ends, I know there's a teammate who will cover any needs that arise. So I don't have to worry about that. This helps me compartmentalize patients and their family members. This creates a clear distinction between my work and my personal life.

★★★

I have strict limits on what I tell patients about my home life. That means staying focused on what my role is, and what my role is not.

★★★

I make sure that my patients know that I'm part of a team. When I emphasize a team concept from the very beginning, patients and family members quickly realize that sometimes I will visit them; but other times, it will be somebody else. I assure them that their level of care will remain consistent. Also, I never give out my phone number.

★★★

I've learned that I can be supportive and personable and still keep my home life private. I know that I can earn a patient's trust without sharing details about my time away from work.

★★★

A close relationship with a patient can still include some distance.

★★★

In the recipe of care giving, I see myself as a utensil, not an ingredient.

★★★

Leadership is an important part of care giving, and good leaders always have boundaries with the people they serve. Since I can't be both a leader and a friend to my patients, I choose to be their leader. I let someone else be their friend.

★★★

I never interact on social media with patients or their families. Because I live in the same community where I work, I might encounter relatives of former patients while I'm out shopping. In my case, it's especially important to keep boundaries.

★★★

I remind myself that it's the patient's journey, not mine.

★★★

I trust in discretion. But I also trust in God, that he will guide me to connect with patients in an appropriate way. Each patient is unique, and each situation is different.

★★★

I've learned to begin, maintain, and end patient relationships with dignity and respect. I do not allow a patient's problem to become my own problem, and I strive to be professional at all times.

★★★

By choice, I do not attend patient funerals. I love my patients when they're in my care; but when the shift ends, I turn them over to God and pray for peace.

★★★

QUESTION: What is the hardest part of your job right now?

A SAMPLE OF RESPONSES

My current challenge is caring for drug and alcohol addicted patients. There's unrest in their spirit and in their life. Loved ones are often angry and hurt. Relationships are strained or broken. Sometimes, family members blame themselves and are consumed by guilt. I know I can't fix these things.

★★★

For me, it's realizing that our government and society do not place enough importance on care for the elderly and sick. It's just the nature of healthcare today.

★★★

It's hard for me to admit that there are things I can't control. Ultimately, death is a personal journey, and most of what unfolds is beyond my control. Patients and family members have their own ideas on the kind of care that's needed. Sometimes, I have to allow them to make poor choices. On one hand, I'm bothered that my recommendations are often ignored. On the other hand, I know that patients have the right to make their own decisions.

★★★

Right now, the hardest part of my job is dealing with unrealistic expectations. They come from patients, families, and even coworkers.

★★★

Recently, a patient of mine revoked hospice services. I felt that I couldn't help him. I felt like I failed him.

★★★

Occasionally I have to deal with patients or families that are truly nasty. They can be disrespectful and rude. I know their behavior is driven by pain, but it's still hard to accept. When I discuss this with them, things might get better for a short time. But soon, their behavior returns to "normal."

★★★

Visiting high-acuity patients, and feeling like I'm always in a rush.

★★★

It's hard for me to greet patients with a smile on the days when everything is going wrong.

★★★

There's a price to pay for having a high caseload. Either I feel rushed, or I have to work past my scheduled hours. Either way, it sparks resentment.

★★★

It isn't easy for me to accept the truth: I have limitations!

★★★

This may sound odd, but I get really frustrated with technological problems such as a computer malfunction or a software glitch.

★★★

I find it difficult to address emergent needs while dealing with the daily demands of my job. I've learned that it's my responsibility to manage this issue. No one else can do it for me.

★★★

QUESTION: What is the most rewarding aspect of your work?

A SAMPLE OF RESPONSES

My work is fulfilling God's purpose for my life, and I am serving his vision. As I ease suffering, I am learning how to die at the same time that I am learning how to live. I feel blessed by the wonderful friendships I've made with coworkers. And finally, I understand how important it is to forgive and to love.

★★★

I know that I'm helping people as they face what may be the most difficult time in their lives.

★★★

It is so rewarding to serve others, to ease their pain and suffering in a small way, even if it's just for a short period of time.

★★★

I have learned so much from my patients. Sometimes I feel that I receive more than I give.

★★★

The most rewarding part of my job is the feeling I get when a patient is finally comfortable. At times, it's like solving a puzzle: *What's causing his agitation?* After I find that missing piece – and the pain, anxiety, and nausea subside – it is so rewarding!

★★★

For me, it's reassuring my patients that their hospice team will be working hard to support them and help manage any pain.

★★★

I am privileged to work with the most amazing people!

★★★

It's satisfying when I'm able to get a family to understand that the journey belongs to their loved one who is dying, not them.

★★★

I am living my purpose for this life!

★★★

I love to witness the peace which comes when a patient has wrestled with impending death, but then is able to accept it. It's very rewarding to help people sustain their spirit in a storm of life that had threatened to overwhelm them.

★★★

When I make post-death phone calls to family members, it's rewarding to hear their gratitude for my help and support.

★★★

I enjoy helping people perceive life differently, and helping them discover ways to cope with seasons of pain, sadness, and hardship.

★★★

It is such an honor to serve at the bedside of a person who is actively dying. I'm especially gratified when my care leads to slower, easier breathing, or results in more relaxed facial muscles — signs that the patient is experiencing greater peace and comfort.

★★★

I know that I'm making a difference, that I'm alleviating someone's suffering.

★★★

Realizing that I'm improving a patient's day. I'm making people feel better than they felt before I arrived.

★★★

QUESTION: What wisdom or advice would you offer to a first-time hospice caregiver?

A SAMPLE OF RESPONSES

First, it's not about you. You may not view someone's passing as a "good death" but the dying process unfolds as it is meant to be. There's a Divine moment to be born, and a Divine moment to die. Since there are no do-overs, each day should be your *best* day. And when you don't have your best day, forgive yourself. Finally, prepare to be changed forever – and for the good!

★★★

Remember to take care of yourself. Otherwise, you won't be able to give your patients 100%.

★★★

A hospice career isn't for everyone, but it's the most rewarding job I've ever had. Sometimes, it is difficult to the point of being impossible. The work will frustrate you, move you, and ultimately make you a better person – if you let it!

★★★

Take time off when you need it. And really listen carefully to your patients and their families to make sure that everyone is sharing the same goals.

★★★

Find out what is important to your patient. Then, be sure your patient knows that his desires are important to you. It is your patient's journey, so let his wishes guide the way.

★★★

There will be good days and bad days. Just hold your head up and breathe deeply. All things shall pass.

★★★

Your patients are likely to be angry at times, and you might become a misdirected target of that anger. So don't take things personally.

★★★

Prepare to be humbled. Be empathetic and compassionate. And take care of yourself, because there will be days when you'll need all the extra love you can give yourself.

★★★

Stay centered and strong in your personal faith, but also be open to new spiritual awakenings. Keep in mind that you are an advocate for the person who is dying, and that might lead to friction with certain family members. Finally, remember that death anxiety is very complex. Ativan doesn't fix everything!

★★★

As you drive home from work, try to clear your mind. Let go of the day's emotional roller coaster. And set aside time each week for fun, recreation, and relaxation.

★★★

From time to time, you may experience something traumatic — something that shatters your confidence or undermines your faith. If this happens, reach out to your supervisor or a trusted colleague. Talk about what happened and share your feelings. Think of it as a debriefing opportunity. But whatever you do, don't keep painful feelings bottled-up inside.

★★★

Build a relationship with God. You will find it helpful in this line of work.

★★★

Each day offers unique opportunities. You will be positioned in strategic places at just the right time to nurture comfort, peace, and hope.

★★★

Let your gifts and talents be evident in your work. Enjoy what you do!

★★★

Surround yourself with positive people who help you grow, make you laugh, and add meaning to your life.

★★★

Patients are not numbers. Always give them the personal dignity and respect they deserve. It's unfair to think that family members can watch the decline or death of a loved one with the same degree of calmness and detachment that you do. Bear in mind that you only see a snapshot of someone's life. So don't project your own experiences or expectations onto the people you're serving.

★★★

Do this work because you care! You won't last if your heart isn't in it. On days off, do things that bring you abundant joy! Be mindful of special moments, and celebrate them – both at work and at home.

★★★

LOST IN A DESERT: A GUIDED IMAGERY

Only in your imagination can things be called beautiful
or ugly, well-ordered or confused. *Baruch Spinoza*

★★★

Begin by taking three deep breaths … Now, imagine falling asleep in your own bed, only to awaken in a vast, barren desert. In every direction, sand stretches farther than your eyes can see, and a blistering sun dominates the cloudless sky. Questions arise. *How did I get here? How could I have wandered so far from the comfort and safety of my home? Why am I suddenly alone, so distant from everyone I love?*

Trying to remain hopeful, you start walking. Something seems familiar, but it isn't the bleak landscape. Rather, it's your feelings of sadness, inadequacy, and frustration that you know so well. They have, it seems, been your closest companions for a long while. As the hours pass, you keep walking. You ignore your parched throat and weary legs. Your mind screams, *Can I get some help? Please God, would that be asking too much?* Yet, part of you feels the sting of guilt; for it's been a long time since you've reached out to your Creator.

The trek across this desolate sea of sand is depleting you. Facing insufferable heat and exhaustion, you wonder if it's possible to take another step. Then, a tiny dot appears on the horizon. You push forward and, getting closer, your spirit soars. *Is there a reprieve from the savage sun? Is it real, or just a cruel mirage?* Getting closer, newfound energy propels you. Now you're practically running, and what you see is hard to believe. A moment later, you're surrounded by lush vegetation. Large palm trees offer merciful shade. Stunned by the tranquil beauty of this sanctuary, you pause and rest. Your eyes are drawn to an array of tropical plants. You are surrounded by vibrant colors and echoing sounds. Exotic birds offer raucous greetings, and playful monkeys chatter in the trees – as if to ask, *Why worry? Why doubt?* Next, you see a pond that's graced by white and pink and yellow lilies. In the midst of an unforgiving desert, you revel in this heavenly oasis.

To your surprise, a gentle rain begins to fall. You stand tall and look skyward with outstretched arms. With an open mouth, your tongue captures enough precious water to quench your burning thirst. In a state of wonder and awe, you close your eyes and bow your head. Immersed in this healing rain, you realize that it's washing away your guilt, your sadness, your frustrations, and your shortcomings. This holy rain is cleansing you of past mistakes and lingering regrets; it's erasing those haunting disappointments and neglected promises. This sacred water is washing away the pain of broken relationships and the suffering of misguided choices.

Finally, the rain subsides. Standing beneath a glorious rainbow, you bathe in sublime light. You feel renewed and replenished, so free of earthly burdens. You sense God's closeness, and know that he's at your side. You realize that God will never abandon you, and that he loves you just the way you are. Then, an epiphany – an understanding that you are worthy of God's love! This awareness is both humbling, and liberating. Now, you feel a profound inner peace. You are whole and joyous! You are safe, and you are loved.

Inspired by Douglas C. Smith

★★★

Closing Reflection ...

Suppose you are lost in a desert and dying of thirst. Then, you find a pump that has one bottle of water next to it. And there's a note: *Prime the pump by pouring the bottled water down the spout. Pump as much fresh water as you wish to drink. Refill the bottle for the next traveler.*

Would you simply drink the life-saving water stored in the bottle and move on? Or would you follow the instructions and pour the bottled water down the spout, hoping that it will prime the pump?

Or think of it this way. Would you choose to save your own life at the expense of the next passerby? Would you be willing to risk your own death by attempting to prime the pump?

★★★

DAY THIRTY

LOOKING BACK, MOVING FORWARD

Not all who wander are lost. *J. R. R. Tolkien*

★★★

Thirty takeaways ...

1. As individual pathways unfold, many travelers – but not all – will become more aware of God's presence and, through Divine grace, they will gain a greater understanding of truth and reality. Try to perceive your life as if it were a challenging, but rewarding, spiritual journey. Then, make a commitment to raise your level of consciousness.

2. Consciousness shapes what you think, what you say, what you do, and what you don't do. Your personal level of consciousness will elevate as you grow in love and faith, and there are countless ways to achieve this outcome, including: prayer, reflection, worship, meditation, and study; and through selfless service; and by offering forgiveness to others and to oneself; and by withholding judgment; and through an open but disciplined mind; and by adhering to a high moral code; and by learning from one's mistakes; and through expressions of praise and gratitude; and by living in the present moment; and by extending genuine respect and heartfelt kindness to everyone you meet, without exception.

3. God *is* love, and Divine love is beyond human comprehension. It is unconditional and freely given. And though you needn't earn God's love, you *are* deserving of it.

4. Your personal journey to discover God's truth and reality cannot be delegated. Moreover, it's a required pilgrimage. Your only choice in the matter is when to begin.

5. Because a large portion of the world's population is functioning at a low level of consciousness, an alarming number of

individuals are angry, self-centered, dishonest, and prone to violent behavior. Despite this, hope and optimism are justified; for consciousness research suggests that, slowly but surely, our planet is becoming a kinder, gentler place.

6. In all matters, the scales of justice are destined to be balanced. Sometimes this reckoning, and the atonement which follows, happens in the here and now. Other times, it occurs in the afterlife. If there were no life after death, then we could rightfully conclude that Divine Order is unfair – and privately wonder if God is merciful.

7. Serving as messengers, guides, comforters, and protectors, angels travel freely among physical and metaphysical domains. Angels are always nearby, ready to gather around you during troubled times. And like the wind, an angel's presence might be something you feel, but not see.

8. Made in God's image, humanity's essence is love. Yet evil is real. Moreover, people can choose to turn their backs to God's grace and mercy; for there are, in fact, eternal realms of darkness, despair, and hopelessness.

9. Spiritual growth not only enlightens the seeker, it uplifts humanity as a whole.

10. In a perfect world, governments would defend, with rigor and resolve, the personal liberty of their citizens and promote equal opportunity for all. And ideally, organized religions would promote respect and tolerance among our diverse nations and cultures. But today's era, in a certain way, resembles those of the past: Everything that bears the mark of human fingerprints is corruptible, including governments and religions.

11. Prayers are powerful. So in the midst of a crisis, find the clarity to say: *God, help me!*

12. Although it is invisible, gravity's force is very real and extraordinarily powerful. In a similar fashion, God cannot be seen; yet Divine love is absolutely real and immeasurably powerful. That said, no amount of evidence can convince people of the truth they do not want.

13. When a belief that's true (for example, the earth revolves around the sun) is compared to an opposing belief that's false (the sun revolves around the earth), and when both views are presented with conviction and authority, the mind is unable to distinguish fact from fiction. This caveat explains why so many people are struggling to recognize reality. Yet, because we are born with this limitation, there's an underlying innocence to our perpetual state of confusion. And when you see the world through a lens of innocence, it's much easier to be empathetic and compassionate. It's much easier to forgive others and oneself.

14. You are immersed in Divine grace. Nevertheless, seasons of hardship will test your patience and trust. So be aware that, while facing adversity, you are not alone.

15. Sacred texts suggest that, similar to a journey on earth, each afterlife experience is one of a kind. Death is the end of one chapter, and the start of a new one — a fresh beginning that is characterized by unbridled promise and limitless possibilities. There's reason to believe that, in the afterlife, you will continue to grow in love and faith. Indeed, there may be opportunities to raise your consciousness to dazzling new heights.

16. Placing the needs of another above the needs of oneself is an expression of love. Yet, caregivers who nurture and look after themselves are better prepared to serve their patients. Or think of it this way: There may be times when you must address personal needs first; for an unhealed healer helps no one.

17. As prompted by human nature, one of our foremost desires is to be safe and loved, especially when we are sick or feeling vulnerable. We also yearn to be part of something greater than ourselves. However, our deepest, innermost desire is to be adored by God.

18. Nature's display of abundance and beauty is a manifestation of God's love.

19. Inner stillness and equanimity promote wellness, including improved physical health. Keep in mind that each morning presents a brand new opportunity to make healthy, life-affirming choices.

20. Fueled by energy, human bodies do what they're designed to do: hearts pump, lungs expand, muscles flex, and joints bend. Bodies are miraculous vessels of life. Yet, while they are amazingly resilient, human bodies are emphatically mortal. In some cases, they succumb to sudden, unexpected trauma. Other times, they slowly grow old, tired, sick, and broken. Either way, flesh and bones are destined to betray you. But like the immortal breath of creation, your spirit – your soul – is impervious to aging and fatigue; spirit is invulnerable to injury, disease, and death.

21. God is always willing to carry the weight of your earthly burdens. And the moment you hand over your problems to God, there's literally nothing left to worry about!

22. Building a relationship requires hard work, and that's why you learn and grow so much from each one. While exploitative relationships may come and go quickly, a relationship founded on love can flourish for a lifetime. Every relationship, regardless of its duration, offers instructive life lessons. And each human interaction holds the potential to be transformative – to be a holy encounter.

23. Humanity continues to grapple with its greatest fears: old age, sickness, poverty, and death.

24. Those who embrace a victim identity hold themselves blameless for the circumstances they face. Lacking a sense of personal accountability and self-determination, victims rarely engage in introspection. What's more, they seldom set goals for themselves. People who cling to victimhood are, in fact, making a destructive, dispiriting, and disempowering choice.

25. As a caregiver, you join with people and walk with them for a short while. You provide comfort and support, and your work is meaningful. But it is their journey, not yours; and it is their pain, not yours. Remember to establish and keep boundaries.

26. Fortunately, there are effective interventions to help you manage anxiety, stress, and burnout. Refer to them often, and use them as needed. Bear in mind that life doesn't always have

to be serious. Try to find reasons to laugh, even if it's laughing at yourself.

27. Make a point to identify things that you are grateful for. Find beauty, discover awe, celebrate abundance, and count your blessings. Then, offer praise!

28. Miracles are happening all around you. On rare occasions, they are loud and grand; but most miracles are quiet and humble: a chance encounter, an unexpected smile, a warm embrace, an act of kindness, or perhaps just a shift in perception. In truth, a miracle is anything that increases your awareness of God's presence.

29. Love is a mystery, an enigma that cannot be fully defined. Nor can love be entirely explained or understood. You know intuitively that love may be predicted, but not controlled or manipulated. You know instinctively that love might be suppressed, but never extinguished. Though it bends, love does not break. Having no true opposite, love unveils the illusion of polarities. Yet, there's a paradox: For love is both the lamb *and* the lion, the rose *and* the thorn, the sweet *and* the bitter.

30. As you form trust-based relationships with your patients, try to envision care giving as a ministry. Then, strive to make it a spirit-guided one. You can start by asking God to use you as an instrument of his will. Ask to be a conduit of Divine light and love. Pray for guidance to always be at the right place at the right time. And pray for inspiration to say and do what is most helpful. Finally, create a sacred space for your patients by keeping a calm, mindful presence that is void of personal agendas. Sacred space is an authentic environment where people feel safe, and where they can share their thoughts and their stories without being judged.

★★★

Moving forward …

Be real and genuine while visiting your patients. Despite their human faults, offer unwavering respect and acceptance. Be confident, yet humble in their presence. Be honest, kind, and compassionate. Lastly, perceive your work as a gift exchange – a balanced care-giving and care-receiving partnership between you and each patient you serve. Know that joyful giving and grateful receiving are gifts of equal value.

★★★

You know all about sadness. It creeps up on you like an evening fog. Find comfort in small things – an unexpected smile, a gentle touch, a heartfelt story. Notice how people's lives are changed by your interactions with them. Listen closely to their expressions of gratitude. Discover laughter through your tears. See the joy of a life well lived. Let go of pain and disappointment. Hold on to peace and contentment. Celebrate your victories, no matter how small they may seem. Carry forward the happy moments. And never let go of the love in your heart.

★★★

Stars and their countless points of light penetrating an immeasurable blackness; the thin line formed by an endless ocean merging with a boundless sky; such wonders are guides to infinity – such phenomena are shepherds to immortality. Indeed, natural beauty triggers thoughts of the supernatural. So this may explain, in part, how spiritual teachers have concluded: Nothing real can be threatened, and nothing unreal can endure; therein lies the peace of God!

Yet, many people fail to see the wisdom expressed by these words. They will say, *What do you mean nothing real can be threatened? That doesn't make sense.* But upon reflection, a deeper question may arise: What is real, and what isn't? It's an innocent query, one that belies the difficult work needed to explore and, ultimately, to find a meaningful answer. For in order to discover what is real, the traveler must embark on a rigorous spiritual journey. And while moving forward on a meandering pathway, the traveler must ...

1. Discard the superficial. This includes taming the ego and limiting one's pursuit of power, wealth, and status.

2. Expose the ephemeral. This includes being aware that everything physical – regardless of size, form, or composition – is temporary; decay has already begun.
3. Dismiss the vulnerable. This includes accepting that a human being is much more than a body.
4. Unmask the illusory. This includes knowing that death is not final.
5. Embrace the intangible. This includes attaching value to the metaphysical. It is understanding that one's spirit is eternal and imperishable. Finally, it is placing one's trust in God.

The courageous travelers who follow these guideposts will be better equipped to recognize reality when they come upon it. Are you willing to do the work? Are you eager to experience the peace of God?

★★★

Closing reflection ...

I am here only to be truly helpful. I am here to represent Him who sent me. I do not have to worry about what to say or what to do, because He who sent me will direct me. I am content to be wherever He wishes, knowing He goes there with me. And I will be healed as I let Him teach me to heal.

ACIM

★★★

POSTLUDE

Writing a book that includes a spiritual dimension has its own peculiar challenges. For instance, there haven't been any recent, breakthrough discoveries related to human spirituality. So today's authors are, for the most part, recycling ancient wisdom by adding a contemporary twist to very old material. Fortunately, there has been remarkable progress in the study of human behavior. The consciousness research of Dr. David R. Hawkins leaps to mind, and that's why I included a brief overview of his work in this book. Hawkins was a true pioneer, an original thinker who understood the human condition – the sublime *and* the ugly.

Still, on the topic of spiritual insights, there's a misguided conclusion I want to address. Allow me to set the stage. Whenever God or afterlife topics come up at a social gathering or in a group conversation, someone will offer a comment such as: *Oh, we just can't be sure about these things. There's no way to find out if God and heaven are real or not.* Here's my personal reaction to a statement like this – although my thoughts usually remain unspoken:

Yes and no. Yes, there's nothing wrong with a dash of skepticism; and yes, people have existential 'Why me?' mysteries that are impossible to solve. But no, you **can** *be absolutely sure of God's existence and the reality of an afterlife. What you're actually saying, my friend, is that you aren't willing to do the work needed to uncover the truth. You don't have enough interest, curiosity, or pain to compel you to find out what is real and what isn't.*

In other words, this type of person simply isn't ready to begin an earnest spiritual journey. It just isn't an attractive choice at this time in his or her life. I know this, because I *was* that type of person. At age 45, I was cynical, confused, and unhappy. Finally, I reached a point where I was determined to discover what life is all about. Misery had triggered a deep, existential yearning. I was determined to know if there is, in fact, a purpose to life. And I wanted to find out, once and for all, if there really is a God.

For the next eight years, I read books like a madman: spiritual and religious books of all faiths; books on physics and metaphysics; thick books and skinny ones; research books and sacred texts; feel-good books and how-to books; plain books and fancy ones.... You get the idea. Much of the material was, for me, so outside-the-box, I could only read for ten minutes at a time. I literally closed my eyes in an attempt to process it. Every conventional paradigm I had embraced and valued – the pursuit of status, wealth, success – was shattered. The work was exhausting!

As my journey continued, I learned the difference between thinking that God *might* be real, and believing that God *is* real. And as my pathway turned inward, a life-changing moment arrived: I came to *know* that God is real. This ultimately fueled my desire to be a hospice chaplain. Looking back, I see how God led me to the right lesson at the right time. I see how God directed me to the perfect teacher at the perfect moment. It was an arduous leg of my ongoing journey, but reaching that particular milestone was exhilarating – and still is!

★★★

As your own spiritual journey unfolds, God will be there for you. He will never give up on you, or abandon you. And yes, God will offer you just the right lesson at just the right time. All you need to do is ask.

★★★

If you're willing to do the rigorous work – willing to explore your spiritual essence and build a trust-based relationship with God – then prepare to receive gifts beyond your wildest dreams.

★★★

This past October, my wife and I traveled to Door County, Wisconsin. We spent the better part of a week in a cozy cottage on the shore of Lake Michigan. The weather was clear and crisp, and the autumn leaves were at their peak color and splendor. We took long walks in the surrounding woods, joined by our Australian Shepherds, Cody and River. It was a glorious time of rest and renewal, and I was reminded of just how important it is to take care of oneself.

After returning home, I took a few minutes to reflect on the role of mindfulness as a means to nurture wellness and harmony. When we choose to live in the present moment, life is more manageable. We're prepared to savor the joyful moments that come our way, and we're less likely to feel overwhelmed during a crisis. Furthermore, mindfulness enhances clarity which, in turn, helps us find better solutions to the problems we face.

After processing this self-evident reality, I wrote the following verses ...

> Though I don't know how far I will travel this path
> I know I can walk it today
>
> I don't know how far I must carry this load
> But I know I can lift it today
>
> Though I don't know how long I will stare into pain
> I know I can face it today
>
> And I don't know how long I'll hold on to my faith
> But I know I can keep it *this* day!

Peace be with you,

John

ACKNOWLEDGMENTS

Thanks to Kent Anderson, CEO of Ohio's Hospice, who conveyed the need for a wellness book written specifically for hospice caregivers.

Thanks to Lisa Balster, Director of Patient and Family Services at Ohio's Hospice of Dayton, for her affirmation and support.

Thanks to Gayle Simmons, Manager of Chaplains at Ohio's Hospice of Dayton, for her encouragement and support.

Thanks to Mary Murphy – nurse, mentor, and past president of Ohio's Hospice of Dayton – for her advocacy and support.

Special thanks to OHOD staff caregivers Dana Datz, Deb Hunter, Rhonda Konicki, Jena Langford, Kristie Lindon, Bonnie Orlins, and Tom Myers for their editorial guidance, and their evaluations of content efficacy.

Special thanks to OHOD staff caregivers who completed the peer insight survey.

ABOUT THE AUTHOR

Since 2009, John has served as a staff chaplain at Ohio's Hospice of Dayton. He has earned an undergraduate degree in music from the University of Cincinnati, Cincinnati, Ohio; a graduate degree in education from Miami University, Oxford, Ohio; and a graduate degree in theology from Liberty Baptist Theological Seminary, Lynchburg, Virginia. John and his wife, Lynn live in Brown County, Indiana with their Australian Shepherds, Cody and River. John is available for spiritual counseling, bereavement support, and caregiver and spiritual wellness workshops. Please visit John's website at johnalove.com or contact him by email at chaplainjohnalove@gmail.com

An expanded edition of John's earlier book, *Fearless Living and Loving: Christian Hope for the Sick and Their Caregivers* can be purchased online at Amazon.com